The Fabulous Woman's Guide Through Cancer

NICOLA BOURNE

Copyright © 2015 Nicola Bourne

ISBN 10: 1514315580
ISBN-13: 978-1514315583

DEDICATION

To my dad

Who is all that I am, and all that I do.

CONTENTS

ACKNOWLEDGMENTS

This book would quite simply not have been possible without Louise Ross, whose support and encouragement has been inspiring. The same goes for my wonderful sister Natalie Viccars, Tom Bourton and Jessica Brookes for their help, support and continued words of wisdom.

All my tutors at the University of Hertfordshire, in particular Dr Rowland Hughes, Dr Patricia Wheeler and especially Simon Vinnicombe whose remarkable teaching has done more for my ability, confidence and journey back to health than I think they will ever truly know.

Emma Lovelock, Alice Roythorne, Harriet Allchin and Rachel Hobbs for being kind enough to share their experiences.

I want to thank Dr AJ Clark, Dr Nicola Fernhead, Dr Charles Wilson and every single wonderful person who works at Addenbrooke's Hospital, Cambridge and the fabulous Georgette Smith. I owe you all my life.

I am lucky to come from a large and supportive extended family that has been heartbreakingly savaged by cancer. I love them all so much and I know that I inherited my ability to fight, survive and reach for the stars from every single one of them.

To my husband and children, without whom nothing would be possible, for they are my heart.

Chapter One

HI, NICE TO MEET YOU

A woman is like a tea-bag.
You never know how strong she is,
until she is in hot water.
- Eleanor Roosevelt

If you are reading this book, the chances are, you are in hot water!

When I found out that I had cancer, I really wanted to read a book that was written by real women, who had really had cancer and could empathise with my situation and truly enlighten me on what was happening and what was to come. Every book I looked at felt like a textbook or a memoir and that really wasn't what I was looking for. I wanted a book that was going to help me understand how cancer was going to impact *my* life and all the things that my life encompasses, like being a wife, mum, work, my social life and so on.

The sorts of questions I had included, "How am I going to tell my children?" "Can we still go on that holiday?" and "Who will look after the children whilst I'm in treatment?" Obviously, I had lots of questions about my condition as well, but I found an abundance of medical information available to answer those questions. All the *life* questions I had were much harder to find answers and advice to.

I set about gathering all the information that I needed (with help from my husband and sister). You learn so much going through the whole process and then think, *'I wish I had known that earlier'*. As I came to the end of my treatment I decided to collate all the information together into a book. I wrote *The Fabulous Woman's Guide Through Cancer* because it is the book that I had wished I had. I hope to help other women by sharing all that I learned. I really hope that you enjoy this book and that you find it helpful, that it brings you help, comfort and maybe even a little inspiration during this particularly trying time.

MOST IMPORTANTLY

Do not read this book thinking, 'Nicola says that I should be doing this or that'. The only thing that you should be worrying about is getting better and getting through this awful time.

This book is designed to help you and offer suggestions but do not look at it as a never ending to-do list.

You will honestly get bored with the amount of times I say in this book **'be kind to yourself'**, and by that I also mean, don't judge yourself or your abilities, and that is something that can never be overstated. As women we naturally expect the best from ourselves at all times but now is not that time.

I remember in the days after coming home from my operation apologising to visitors about the state of the house. What was I thinking? I had just endured a twelve-hour operation, as if hovering was going to be top of the list for anyone! A friend said to me "I've come to see you, not to check if you've bleached the loo." If your visitors don't see it that way, more fool them.

YOU AND THIS BOOK

I have written this book purposefully so that you can dip in and dip out, reading the sections that are relevant to you, so don't feel you have to read it all in one go – although you obviously can if you would like to. Take what you need from the book, when you need it.

Plus, if like me cancer and all the necessary drugs have zapped your concentration, it can be difficult to take in copious amounts of information, which is why I have tried to keep everything in easy, bite-size chunks.

For these reasons, I have repeated some information to make sure that you don't miss anything, so don't worry if you see the same piece of information twice, it is supposed to be there.

To make it easy for you to navigate I have included the contact details you may need as I mention them in the book and then again under useful contacts at the end of every chapter, so you should always have all the information that you need to hand.

Whatever the suggestion in this book, I would always speak with your oncologist before doing or changing anything to make sure they are happy.

The quote at the beginning of the chapter by Eleanor Roosevelt seemed to follow me around when I had cancer. It was on the chalkboards in coffee shops, quoted in magazine articles, literally all over the place.

Every time it made me smile to myself, reminding me what I was doing and that I *did* have an inner strength that I didn't know I had before cancer. That does not mean it wasn't hard and that there weren't times that I wanted to give up because believe me there were but when all is said and done you have to keep getting up and moving forward and do not let anything stand in your way.

MY STORY

I knew that I had cancer. I had a strong inner feeling and I simply *knew*. I found out that I had bowel cancer when I was 31 and had just given birth to my second child. I was experiencing textbook symptoms and had a basic knowledge of bowel cancer based on a strong family history – my mother died from bowel cancer when she was only 52, after having bowel cancer for the first time five-years earlier. My grandmother also died of bowel cancer in when she was only 69. Even so, getting diagnosed was not as easy as it should have been.

I had been getting rectal bleeding on and off for years. Over the years, I had visited various GPs but they always said the same thing, that I was too young to have bowel cancer, that it was probably a small internal cut and if the bleeding went, there was nothing to worry about. The bleeding *would* stop, so, as far as the GPs were concerned, that was the end of that.

I now know that the bleeding was polyps in the colon, which can bleed intermittently, and it is these polyps that can grow into cancerous tumors. Now I know this was the beginning and could have probably been dealt with in the early stages if my initial concerns and symptoms had been taken seriously.

During my second pregnancy, the bleeding became intolerable but even so my GP still refused to send me for tests. At my post-natal six-week check with the GP, after an unacceptable amount of ridicule for suggesting something could be seriously wrong, I pushed and pushed until finally the GP agreed to refer me for a flexible sigmoidoscopy (a camera in the rectum) which is as pleasant as it sounds! That said, I remember thinking it would be the worst thing in the world but now I know there are much worse things, everything in perspective!

At the end of the procedure, the consultant told me that, yes, he suspected it was cancer. I was immediately referred for CT, MRI and PET scans, which showed the cancer was far more spread than the doctors initially thought. It was at this point that I went into shock.

I found out that the cancer had spread outside the tumor, throughout the whole area and was as far spread as it could be without touching another major organ. I found out that the effected area was so large that I was going to need three-months of chemotherapy and thirty sessions of radiotherapy before they could even operate and then another three-months of chemotherapy afterwards. I found out I would need a twelve-hour operation to remove most of my large intestine, the surrounding tissue and muscles as well as the back of the cervix and because the surgery was so extensive I would need a specialised plastic surgeon to do reconstructive surgery to put me back together again. I found out I would need a permanent colostomy bag which was actually the hardest part for me. I found out that I would be infertile and go into early menopause. I found out I would barely be able to look after my six-month old daughter and two-year old son. That's a lot to find out!

Armed with all this information I began to fight for my life. *The Fabulous Woman's Guide Through Cancer* is what I learnt along the way.

Chapter Two

FRIENDS, FAMILY & HOME

Life is not about waiting for the storm to pass,
it's about learning to dance in the rain.
- Vivian Green

Telling your family and friends can be a difficult part of cancer and can create challenges and unexpected issues. If you have children or people who depend on you, this can be even more difficult. Getting your own mind around what is happening can be hard enough. When you add thinking about telling others and getting organised for everything that is coming… It can all be a lot to do and think about.

TELLING FRIENDS AND FAMILY

I am the sort of person who likes to talk things over. The more I talk something over, the easier it is to gather my thoughts together. When I found out I had cancer, I was more than happy to call friends and family to let them know what was happening to me and have the opportunity to talk it though again and again. I called my closest friends and family the evening I found out and the rest I called over the coming days.

Having said that, it has to be what works best for you. I know other women who couldn't face everyone's reactions or retelling the story over and over again.

Here Emma explains why she chose to tell everyone by email when she found out she had breast cancer.

I couldn't handle dealing with everybody's reactions when I was still trying to deal with my own reaction but I also didn't want to bump into people in the street or at the school gates and have an awkward conversation about what I was going through when they had no idea.

I decided that sending an e-mail was a good way to tell people in one big swoop, especially if I wasn't as close to them. Someone did think the e-mail was a joke though, so I would reconsider my wording if I were to do it again.

Emma, Breast Cancer, 27

If you don't want to tell people yourself you can ask a close family member or friend to call on your behalf. You may consider emailing or texting. Include in your message why you couldn't face telling everyone, they are sure to understand and if they don't, that's their issue, not yours!

If you are thinking about telling people over a period of time, consider people you may bump into, or people that may see each other - would you be happy for them to tell each other? If not remember to ask your friends to keep it quiet until you have had a chance to tell everyone you would like to, or make sure you tell people who are in the same circles at similar times.

THE STUPID THINGS PEOPLE SAY

I would prepare yourself for when people say (what I think) are *very* stupid things. The most common comment being "I knew someone who had cancer and died." Seriously, who are you helping when you say that? There is also my personal favourite, "Just think positively and you'll be fine." Don't get me wrong, positivity is great and *positively* encouraged, but cancer is a little more complicated than just thinking it away. Cancer is not purely a mental test with your survival the prize. But people will tell you to be positive… a lot!

Generally, people love to compare your cancer to someone else they know who had cancer. It may not even be the same cancer or anything like your illness but some people will still compare them. Sometimes I would be told the strangest things like, "At least they caught it early." No they didn't – why are you assuming that?

I think this is usually because people make assumptions based on a previous experience they've had with someone else. This used to drive me mad and annoyingly it's not just with diagnosis, it will be with every stage of your cancer care. I used to get people making assumptions when it came to my colostomy all the time. I was told from the outset that as I was having the sphincter muscle removed, there was absolutely no way it could be reversed. Yet people used to tell me all the time about someone they knew who had it reversed, so they were sure I could get mine reversed too. No amount of me explaining that they could probably have it reversed because they didn't have certain muscles removed, which I have, would convince them that it could never be the case with me.

You may find that you end up consoling the person you have just told rather than the other way around. Personally, I didn't mind this, I actually started becoming quite offended if people didn't need consoling - didn't they care? Obviously, they did, presumably they were holding it together so as not to upset me – right? But seriously, I can certainly see how upsetting it could be if you are struggling with your own emotions and then having to take on someone else's crushed feelings.

Whatever someone's reaction, remember that most people are trying their best. They are not trying to annoy you, they are probably just at a loss for what to say and feel that they need to say something, *anything*.

If someone does say something that offends or upsets you, remember you are in an emotionally raw place. It would be normal to take things to heart that would usually not be such a big deal to you. This is entirely natural so do not feel bad about it. If someone is comparing your cancer to someone else, you could say, there are so many variations (even within the same cancer) they really aren't comparable. Where possible, try to distance yourself from those comments and if someone is upsetting you, maybe mention that you are trying your best to handle it your way... and get them off the phone.

LET PEOPLE HELP, THEY WANT TO

Going from the role of a self-sufficient woman to someone who needs help can be a difficult one. So many people offered to help me at the beginning but I never really knew what, "Let me know if there is anything I can do," meant and I wasn't sure if they were saying it to be polite. I hated the thought of being an imposition on people (apart from my dad and sister – poor them).

Harriet also felt this way saying:

I'd always been very independent and found it difficult to accept help as I felt I was being a burden. I soon learnt that the support I was given by friends and family was their way of coping and made them feel better to be able to do something practical to ease my pressure. I look back now and I don't know what I would have done without them, my illness would have been much harder to manage. Their company used to lift my mood and enabled me to catch up on the latest gossip and keep me distracted from focusing on the sadness I felt at times. Allow people to help you.

Harriet, Bowel Cancer, 39

When I was having chemotherapy, I found eating difficult but needed to increase my vitamin and mineral intake. I asked a family friend if she could make me some chicken soup – but only if it wasn't too much trouble and only if she had time and not to worry at all if she couldn't, I really wouldn't mind. She turned up about four hours later with the biggest tupperwear of chicken soup you have ever seen, telling my husband when she dropped if off that it was so wonderful to know that she could do something to help.

That was when I got it. People aren't just offering on a whim, they care and want to do something to help. They were just waiting for me to tell them what I needed.

Think about what people can do to help you. If you have a friend who loves hunting out deals online, ask them to find you the best... whatever you need. A friend who likes cooking, get them baking your favourite dishes. You will be back and forth to hospital more times than you can imagine, ask different friends to give you lifts.

To help me, I asked friends to post me a copy of their favourite film so I would have lots to watch whilst bed-bound.

Your friends and family will like knowing they are in even a very small way, doing something to help you.

WORKING LIFE

If you can continue to work whilst being treated for cancer will vary massively on your type of cancer and the course of treatment you will be having, as will your desire to continue working. Some people relish continuing work as it gives them a sense of normality in a crazy time, others can't do it with so much happening.

I was a stay-at-home mum when I was diagnosed and told from the outset that my treatment plan was going to mean that I would be too sick to care for the children on my own. It was a devastating blow, but my doctor really was right. I couldn't have done it on my own.

I found that if I stayed at home and rested completely for the first couple of days after being given chemotherapy that I would feel slightly better towards the end of the week and be able to do a few things.

However, if I tried to do too much straight after chemotherapy, it would knock me back and I would be struggling for the rest of week. So for me, it really was best to not do anything those first few days. I appreciate that chemotherapy effects people in different ways but I think this is common for most ladies with cancer.

Telling Your Boss

How your boss or company will handle this kind of news will inevitably vary, as will your company's policy on long-term sickness, as will your ability to continue your job, as will your desire to continue working, and so it goes on....

The one thing I do know is that there are going to be difficulties and changes that you and your employer are going to need to allow for, such as the never-ending appointments, scans and the treatment itself. Depending slight on your treatment plan, you probably won't be able to get better and work to your normal capacity during parts of your treatment, if not all of it.

The one good thing about having cancer (yes I did really did just say that), is that people *tend* to react sympathetically, so hopefully your work will do what they can to support you and they will allow you to take a step backwards or sideways for a while but as I said so much comes down to you and your employer.

REMEMBER

Legislation protects you from being treated unfairly at work because of cancer. If you live in England, Scotland or Wales, the Equality Act 2010 protects you.

The Disability Discrimination Act 1995 and its extension, the Disability Discrimination Order of 2006, protects you if you live in Northern Ireland.

This legislation doesn't just protect employees. It also protects job applicants and people who are self-employed.

If you need legal advice, you should contact a solicitor but if you would like more information with where you stand legally with long term illness Macmillan have a really good leaflet *'Your Rights at Work When You Have Cancer'* that you can download from their website, www.macmillan.com so do take a look. It also has information that you may need about long-term statutory sick pay.

I'm Self-Employed

Well the good news is that your boss should understand about you missing work for an appointment! The bad news is that people who work for themselves are often quite hard on pushing themselves forward, cancer or no cancer.

> ### REMEMBER
> *You do still have rights, even if you are self-employed.*

You may still be entitled to statutory sick pay so you should still have a look at MacMillan's, *'Your Rights at Work When You Have Cancer'* leaflet. www.macmillan.com

HELP! I NEED SOME MONEY

From my experience, getting cancer is an expensive business. The cost of childcare, getting to and from the hospital, parking, everything is just so bloody expensive!

I remember before I had cancer my husband and I were looking at life insurance and I said, 'I'm a stay-at-home-mum, I don't earn any money so I don't need any insurance'. Turns out, it costs thousands to pay someone to do what I do. Actually, it's only part of what I do – lazy nanny didn't work evenings or weekends!

Financial Assistance

Unfortunately the pot for financial assistance was small before we lived in government austerity measures and it appears to be getting even smaller now. The best thing to do is contact your local cancer centre (details about where you can find your local cancer centre are given below) as some of them have in-house financial assistants who know the ins and outs of what is available and for whom. This can be done over the phone by your next of kin if you are not feeling up to it. Once they have all your information they will be able to work out what (if anything) you are entitled to.

TOP TIP

Some hospitals have drastically reduced parking costs for oncology but in my experience the hospitals don't advertise this fact massively, so make sure you ask at your hospital reception to see what you are entitled to.

YOUR LOCAL CANCER CENTER

Most areas have an NHS or charity funded cancer centre. They can be a fantastic resource so I strongly encourage you to find yours. I had my cancer treatment in a different area to where I live, so I actually had access to both and they were very different in the ways that they operated but equally fantastic.

Cancer centres offer services for cancer patients and their primary carers such as:

❖ Counselling
❖ Complementary therapies
❖ Support – emotional and practical
❖ Information

❖ Coffee mornings
❖ Someone you can talk to about any practicalities like financial assistance, benefit entitlement – and if they don't, they should be able to point you in the direction of someone who can.
❖ Some cancer centres offer additional services such as yoga, craft sessions and workshops.

These services are usually offered free or for a heavily reduced rate for the cancer patient and their primary carer. It is honestly worth taking advantage of these fantastic services.

For some unknown reason I felt really embarrassed to use my cancer centres services at first. It was actually my husband who rang and arranged for the two of us to go in and see what was available. Once I had been there and seen how lovely everyone was and how incredible it felt to talk to people who truly understood what I was going though, in a 'we are here for you' capacity as apposed to a medical capacity. I found cancer centres to be truly special places that I needed at the time.

How Do I Find My Local Cancer Centre?

Ask anyone who is involved in your treatment - I am confident they will know. I was given the details of my local cancer centre from my daughter's health visitor, and again from my oncology nurse.

The other centre I used was found through the unbelievable number of leaflets and posters that were located around the oncology suite. So keep your eyes peeled and if you aren't sure, just ask your point of contact in your oncology team.

Failing that Google your area + cancer centre and hopefully one nearby you should come up.

THE INTERNET, FRIEND OR FOE?

I understand the temptation to Google every part of your illness and treatment, honestly I do. You will have so many questions and the answers seemingly at your fingertips. There is a time and a place for the Internet, but I don't believe this is it. Just like during any period of fear or uncertainty is probably not the best time. My advice would be, think about the kind of person you are.

I know I am the kind of person who is going to get upset and stressed by negative comments I read and I would barely register the positive ones. I knew it was best for me not to look. Instead my husband and sister surfed the internet (constantly at the beginning) and slowly filtered relevant pieces of information to me, skipping the irrelevant parts and only giving me truly useful information as and when I needed it. This saved an overwhelming influx of information and this strategy worked really well for me.

INTERNET SEARCHING TIP
FROM MY HUSBAND

You can use the search engine 'Google scholar' to search for technical, in-depth information published by surgeons and oncologists directly, from throughout the world.

Other people need to go into the whole situation knowing absolutely every possibility and possible outcome - the good, the bad and the ugly! As I said before, I understand this, truly, I do.

It gives you a chance to prepare, limit unexpected surprises and explore all possible eventualities. As long as you are able to sift through and find websites and blogs that are relevant and well balanced, you should be able to find all the information you are looking for.

REMEMBER

People are more likely to go online and complain than they are to go online to write about how successful and fabulous their operation / treatment / doctor was. If you are only reading horror stories, it is going to be scarier and give a distorted view of what's happening.

It is also worth bearing that in mind if you are not able to find many positive stories, it doesn't mean they don't exist, it may just mean no one has written one yet.

To Share or Not to Share

Many of us are used to sharing every aspect of our lives on social media now, but when are we over sharing? Strangely, this seems to be something that people who don't have cancer have an opinion on. Only *you* can decide if you want to share having cancer on social media.

I did share. I didn't write, "Hey everyone I have cancer!" but once most people knew about it, I would occasionally post something like "Last day of chemotherapy, yay" or even "Struggling a bit today, please send some support" and so many people would write the kindest things which gave me a bit of an emotional lift.

As much as I didn't mind the initial ring round, I didn't want to be calling people every five minutes letting them know how I was getting on. Social media (with privacy settings) was a great way of giving people a general idea of how I was doing and as a lot of my family live in the USA it was a great way of keeping them updated.

I will always remember the time when one of my uncles in Texas changed his profile picture to a picture of him and I and encouraged everyone to do the same, as a sign of support and solidarity. I woke up in the middle of the night feeling nauseous and so sorry for myself and when I looked at my phone and there were all these pictures of me in my timeline with words of love. I was so touched. Such a simple thing, but in that moment it really lifted me and made me smile.

Here Rachel talks about why she decided not to share any details about her bowel cancer on social media:

> *I decided early on that I would prefer not to talk about my cancer openly on social media and asked my close friends and family to also respect my wishes and message me privately about anything related to my illness. I wanted to protect myself, and my loved ones, from the inevitable 'charitable' looks and awkward silences when out and about. I didn't want to become 'the one with cancer' topic of conversation for old friends and acquaintances. I knew that well-meant comments about 'someone else's Granny having that and she's fine now!' weren't going to help!*
>
> *Rachel, Colorectal Cancer, 37*
> *Secondary Colorectal Cancer in Lungs, 39*

RELEASE YOUR INNER MISS MONEYPENNY

There is an old saying, '*Hope for the best. Plan for the worst,*' and this couldn't be truer than when you have cancer.

If you are a born organiser, this will probably be second nature to you. If you are like me, it's not! Either way, I would advise you to release your inner Miss Moneypenny and get the administration side of things organised to make life easier down the line.

Start Filing

The amount of information, appointment letters, telephone numbers, details and bits of paper you are given when finding out you have cancer can be overwhelming. Even if that filing system is one large folder that the many pieces of paper can be chucked into, start filing. I had a large lever-arch file with sections, which I split into:

- ❖ Appointment letters
- ❖ Diagnosis letters
- ❖ Follow up letters
- ❖ Scan results
- ❖ Treatment information
- ❖ Surgery details
- ❖ Post-care details
- ❖ Miscellaneous

This way all papers remained relatively organised and if I needed to locate something, I had a good idea where it would be. It also came in handy if someone else had to find something for me or file something away.

Fridge Details

It is definitely worth getting a list up on the fridge of all your medical details. That way, if there is an emergency and someone needs to phone on your behalf, they can easily find the necessary details. Plus, it will save you rooting around if you needed to call your doctor quickly. I would include:

- ❖ Your NHS number
- ❖ Hospital number
- ❖ Hospital telephone number, address and person of contact
- ❖ Hospital doctors names and jobs
- ❖ Your GP's name, address and telephone number
- ❖ Emergency contact details such as your husband, best friend, etc.
- ❖ Contact details of anyone who is looking after your children such as a nanny or childminder plus or their school or nursery
- ❖ Contact details of emergency person/s who can look after your children in an emergency

TOP TIP

The job of collating all the information and typing it up could be given to a friend who wants to do something to help.

First Aid Kit

I am sure your oncologist will have explained this but when you start treatment, in particular chemotherapy, illness can come on very quickly and can be particularly dangerous.

It is very important that you don't get a temperature when you are having chemotherapy so it is good to have a first aid kit handy with:

- ❖ A thermometer
- ❖ Painkillers (always check your temperature before taking paracetamol as it will lower your temperature meaning that a thermometer wont give an accurate reading and if you have a high temperature you need to call your oncology team immediately)
- ❖ Any side-effect medication

If you do have a temperature you MUST contact your oncologist immediately, but I am sure they will explain that to you.

All these bits, together with anything else you need on a regular basis, together with your fridge details should mean that you are covered in case of an emergency.

USEFUL CONTACTS

www.cancerresearchuk.org
www.macmillan.org.uk

Chapter Three

WHAT ABOUT THE CHILDREN?

Start where you are. Use what you have.
Do what you can.
- Unknown

Having children adds a difficult dimension to an already difficult situation. I experienced a complete mix of emotions with regards to the children when finding out I had cancer. My son was two-years-old and my daughter, a tiny three-months-old when I was diagnosed.

This created the hardest part of having cancer for me, both logistically and emotionally but at the same time my children were the force that kept me strong and helped get me through the darkest of days. As their mum I wanted to protect them from the realities of cancer, not force them to face it head on. How to handle the finer points was a continual worry for me. Whether it is your child, grandchild, niece or friend, it can be very difficult talking to children about cancer.

How you tell a child will vary, depending on their age. The most important thing is that you speak to them in a language they understand. My daughter was only three-months-old so she definitely didn't have a clue that anything was going on. My son had just turned two when I was diagnosed and had no real understanding of serious illness or of what cancer was at the beginning. As the year went on and his understanding increased so we tried to continue building on what he already knew.

As my daughter still had a health visitor at the time, I was able to speak with her about how to talk with children about serious illness. Thankfully she was able to give me plenty of advice, most of which is included below:

TELLING TODDLERS

Toddlers believe that they are the center of the universe. As far as they are concerned no world exists beyond them so when something *does* go wrong, they think that it is their fault. That is why it is vitally important that you don't just assume they are too young to understand. They are very perceptive and they will know that something is up, so you need to say something rather than trying to brush things under the carpet.

A Few Tips

- ❖ Speak to the child in a language they will understand. Whichever words you use to describe when they aren't well, use that wording. We explained it to my son as; 'Mummy has an oowee in her tummy.'
- ❖ Toddlers learn with all their senses and tend to be very visual so show them as much as you can, as well as talking to them. After the operation, I was able to show my son my scars so that he could visualise mummy's oowee, which helped him to understand.
- ❖ TV shows on channels such a Cbeebies often have segments when a child visits a hospital to get better or showing what it is like to be a doctor. Watch these shows with your child, pointing out the different people involved including the doctors, nurses, families and patients. Your child can then relate back to this information to help them understand what happens when you go to hospital.

TELLING CHILDREN

As a child's understanding is greater, so probably will be their fears. Once again, speak to them in the language they use. Children tend to respond better to heavy conversations when doing something they want to be doing. If they like drawing or football, discuss things whilst they are drawing or while playing football with them. I find that my son is usually happy to have a chat when we are in the car together so going for a drive was always a good time to talk to him.

When it comes to school age children, there is the possibility of them hearing things in the playground. Ask them if their friends have said anything because if you know what they are being told by school friends, it will give you a chance to respond. Keep talking to them about their fears, however trivial or obvious the answers may seem to you.

If there are specifics you do not want the children to hear about in the playground, you could ask your friends not tell their children those specific points, but I think this is always going to be difficult. A child may overhear something and get the wrong end of the stick and before you know it it's around the playground like Chinese whispers. It may simply be easier to make sure children are already armed with all the information they may need if their friends bring it up.

This was something that Rachel thought about when talking about her cancer with her son and friends explaining:

I was as honest with him as you can be with my son and talked about Mummy's strong medicine through a tube and needing to have lazy days in bed to have a rest and get better. I wanted the information he heard to come from us, not children in the playground who'd heard via their parents. I had already asked my friends and family to respect my wishes and message me privately about anything related to my illness so that I could protect my son from here-say and miss information.

Rachel, Colorectal Cancer, 37
Secondary Colorectal Cancer in Lungs, 39

When my son was around four and needed to visit the doctor and he was panicking. Eventually I realised what was going on when he asked if he was going to have to go to hospital for a long time like I did. At this point I decided to tell him that I had an illness called 'cancer,' which was very serious and it took a long time for the doctors to make it better, but they did and I am completely fine now.

I also made it clear that he did *not* have cancer only a cough (or whatever it was) and that he just needed a little bit of medicine from the GP. Now he can actually call 'cancer' by its name, it seems to have made it easier for him to distinguish between cancer and just being a little bit unwell.

TELLING TEENAGERS & YOUNG ADULTS

In writing this segment, I speak from further personal experience, having been the twenty-two year old daughter of a *fabulous* woman with bowel cancer.

My mother always wanted to protect us children and did not want to expose us to the harsher realities of cancer. I can honestly say that one of the worst things is feeling that you do not fully understanding what is going on, or feeling like you are being kept out of the loop.

As a mother, I understand the want to protect your children from all things frightening but if they are teenagers or older, they will not appreciate it. Be as honest with them as possible. Where possible, let them be involved, let them help you. No doubt you have spent *years* taking care of them, let them take care of you for a change! It will give them a sense of purpose and relieve the frustrating sense of impotence which many loved ones may feel standing on the sidelines.

With teenagers, the whole center of the universe thing may not have disappeared yet so be specific about how they can help you. Even when you aren't a teenager it can be hard to second guess what people need at a time like this so don't expect them to know, give them a hand and really spell it out for them.

COPING SUGGESTIONS

When you are a mum, I know your default mode is to be superwoman. To fight cancer, be the best mother in the world and be a present parent for your child. That was certainly what I was aiming for initially.

What I learnt over time was that I don't think you can fight cancer and be an ever-present, best mum – well, I'm sure you are the best, but maybe not in the all-encompassing way you envisioned before you had cancer. I had such a clear idea what I thought motherhood was going to be and cancer was robbing me of it. It is a hard concept to get your head round, there are no two ways about it.

I know that there is no *good* time to have cancer, but having small children, I felt it was particularly unfair. I felt like I missed most of my daughters first year. After getting to spend every moment with my son when he was a baby, this was really difficult for me. I missed the first time my daughter rolled over and sat up, the nanny we were forced to hire enjoyed these moments.

I will always remember fondly my fabulous nanny telling me that while I was at a chemotherapy appointment, my daughter stood up and lifted her leg as if to take her first step, so our nanny quickly pushed her over before she could and carried her around for the rest of the day so I wouldn't miss it – bless! Of course my daughter didn't try walking again for another couple of weeks but I was there to see it (yay).

As with all these things, you just attempt to maintain something that resembles a balance. It is a constant and evolving situation as your health and ability dips and strengthens throughout so you just keep trying.

Here are a few things that I found help me through the constant changes:

Keep Things in Perspective

When I used to get upset about not being with the children for certain things, my husband used to say; "The children don't care if you see them roll over for the first time or not, they care that you are alive, to be with them and watch them grow up." Now, aint that the truth! I used to try to keep that in mind when I felt I was missing out because it's so true.

Carve Out Some Special Time

When I was having chemotherapy or was bed bound, I used to get the children into my bed and read them their bedtime story. Or go and snuggle up with them on the sofa whilst they had TV time.

All children love routine so if there is one part of the day, no matter how tiny, that they can know you will be involved in, I think it works quite well.

Bonds Are Built on More Than Time

The bond with my daughter was something I worried about, as she was only three-months-old when I was diagnosed. When you are pregnant you are told about all these things you *have* to do with your baby, otherwise you are basically stamping all over their childhood and any chance of you bonding with each other, but it's simply not true. My daughter and I have a wonderful bond. We love each other eternally and no amount of me being in hospital and chemotherapy has changed any of that.

Plus you are going through their childhood with a determination to live for them that most other parents will sympathise with hypothetically, but will never actually experience.

So don't panic if you aren't around as much as you planned, because I am confident your bond will still be the same.

MOST IMPORTANTLY
Give yourself a break and just enjoy all the moments that you can.

CHILDCARE

If you need help with childcare there are a number of options you can consider, with pros and cons to all of them. It is about finding one that works best for you and your family, when taking into account your lifestyle, illness, family routine, how much help you are going to need, what you can afford and so forth. There is so much to think about when it comes to childcare, hopefully some of the information below will help.

TOP TIP

When meeting potential childcare providers, I think the best advice I can give you is to go with your gut. You are their mum and you know what is going to work best for you all. I have been to places that have been awarded an 'outstanding' Ofsted rating but they aren't the right setting for my children.

You get a feel for a place or a person and you will know when you are in the right place or with the right person.

Help from Friends and Family

PROS: Friends and family can be an amazing help. People close to you will probably want to help and this is a fantastic way to get everyone involved. It means that the children can have fun hanging out with different members of the family and friends and it can be nice for you to have them around. It is also usually free! Essentially it is just so much nicer having someone you love and trust in your home when you are in such a vulnerable place emotionally and physically.

CONS: It can require a lot of organisation, making

sure the right people are always in the right place at the right time and that they all know the children's routines. It can also be difficult to tell people what to do when they are doing you a favour. My dad used to joke, "As long as they are alive." My response – "Not really!" I have routines and a structure that I wanted to try to retain, especially as the cancer period is going on for so long. If my daughter oversleeps during her afternoon nap she won't go down in the evening and it's my husband or I who are up all night with her, not the cheeky person who let her oversleep! I can say that to my dad but I personally would find it harder to be so honest with other members of the family or friends.

Hire a Nanny

PROS: Having one person look after your children can offer good continuity of care. Nannies work in your home and replace the mother's role during working hours. This means that, as well as looking after the children they will also cook for the children, wash their clothes, keep their bedroom, any play areas and toys clean and tidy, all of which can be immensely useful. They can take and collect children from school, classes, keep any existing playdates and maintain friendships with other children.

The fact that they will be looking after your children in your home can be an upside or downside depending on how you look at it. My nanny was a little superstar and on chemotherapy weeks would make sure the children were out of the house at the park or on playdates. I liked having the children at home so I could pop down and see them whenever possible and then head back upstairs when I needed to.

Nannies are not legally required to be Ofsted registered but you can ask for them to be (it would be common for you to cover the cost of them becoming Ofsted registered if it was something you wanted them to do) but they should be qualified, CRB checked and have their own insurance.

CONS: The cost! Nannies can cost a small fortune. The exact amount varies depending on where in the country you are based, but if they are working full-time, they need a full-time wage which can be anything between £20000 and £30000 per annum, sometimes more if they have extensive experience.

If your nanny is off sick, you wont have anyone else to look after your child. Your nanny is entitled to annual leave and should their holiday coincide with a time when you need help, you would need to arrange alternative care.

Consider a Nanny Share

PROS: One option to help reduce the cost is a nanny share. The nanny looks after your and someone else's children and the cost is split between both families.

CONS: The downside of a nanny share is that there may be times when you have another child or children in your house when you are not feeling well, but you would be able to arrange all the details between you, the nanny and the other family, maybe ensuring the children are looked after at the other family's home during difficult weeks.

Knowing friends who have done this, here are a few things to think about and discuss with the other family:

❖ *Annual Leave*

You may not be interested in going on holiday but the other family might. If so, they may want the nanny to take holiday at the same time. How would that suit you? What arrangements would you need to make over that period?

❖ *Sick Leave*

If your nanny is off sick, will you be responsible for looking after both sets of children or just yours?

❖ *Expenses*

Would you have a joint account and agree on amounts you would pay at the beginning of the week? Travel expenses?

❖ *Classes and Groups*

What if they would like their child to go to a particular class that you don't want to pay for or visa-versa?

Using a Childminder

Childminder's look after a number of children in their home and you would usually drop your child off and collect them at set times.

PROS: A real benefit is that it should feel like a home away from home. There will be other children there so your child will benefit from the social interaction with others, but never too many since childminder's are only allowed a certain number of children at any one time.

They may be able drop off and collect children from school, depending on existing commitments.

Childminder's should be qualified, CRB checked and insured. It is a legal requirement that childminder's are Ofsted registered and that their homes are kept to the standard required by Ofsted. It is also a legal requirement that any other adults who may be in the home at the same time as your children, (such as their partner or children over the age of sixteen) have to be CRB checked.

CONS: If the childminder is ill, who will step in and watch the children? I have actually experienced a couple of times when my childminder's own children were off school sick meaning that she couldn't look after my son on those days.

The children may have to take part in some of the errands the childminder needs to run so I would check if that is something that they would need to do and if you are comfortable with your children going along for the ride.

You may not always feel well enough to drop off and collect your children from the childminder, so you may need to think about who would drop them off and collect them for you.

WHEN LOOKING FOR A CHILDMINDER
Recommendations are always best, so if you know of anyone who already uses a childminder, and assuming that they are happy with the childminder, ask them for their details.

The cost of a childminder does vary hugely based on where you live. I used to pay £7 per hour but a friend who lives 25 minutes drive away pays £4.50. Best to ask around and see what the local rate is.

Nursery

When I first had children I was so confused between nursery schools, preschools, nursery classes, so many options! The nurseries I am talking about are the day nurseries that take children between 6 months and 5 years old. They are normally open all day, sometimes from 7am to 7pm for working mums and dads.

PROS: They usually have a number of rooms that are broken down into age groups and your child will be in a room with their peers.

Nurseries are legally required to be Ofsted inspected and have a certain number of employees for the number of children they take.

A really good thing about nursery is that you never need to worry about someone phoning in sick. They will arrange their staff throughout the different rooms to make sure that all the children can still get into nursery, which is a great thing for you not to need to worry about.

CONS: The downside of covering sickness and holiday can be that the nursery staff may move around rooms quite a bit to keep the ratio of staff to child correct. If your child is like my son and prefers consistent care, this can be unsettling, but if your child is like my daughter, this won't faze them at all. Different nurseries operate in different ways so it is worth asking when you go to visit.

USEFUL QUESTIONS TO ASK

When looking at nurseries, childminder's or hiring a nanny, there can be a lot to think about.

Here are a few questions to help you get the most out of your visits with them:

- ❖ Have you looked after children in my child's age group before?
- ❖ How do you discipline bad behaviour? Can you give examples?
- ❖ Can you keep a diary with photos?
- ❖ When did you last do a first aid course? What would you do if my child started choking?
- ❖ How would you keep a two-year-old busy if the weather was bad outside and they were bored?
- ❖ What sort of meals do you cook? Have you cooked for toddlers/children before? What will you do if they don't eat? Can you make a meal plan for the week?
- ❖ What will happen if someone is / you are off sick?
- ❖ For a nanny or childminder – will you retain the friendships, classes or groups the children are already involved in?

TOP TIP

If your child will be experiencing a combination of childcare providers it can be nice to give them a visual plan for the week.

Have a large sheet of paper split into days and I stick a picture of who would be looking after him on that day underneath. It allowed him to feel a little more certain of where he was going and whom he was going to be with.

HIRING A NANNY

With nurseries or childminder's, you pick the place or person, send your child and get invoiced. Everything is, more or less, arranged for you. When hiring a nanny there is actually quite a lot for you to do, as you have to become their employer.

How to Find a Nanny

I think when looking for a nanny, it is best to speak to someone for a recommendation. I found mine by asking a friend who is a nanny where she found her placement and she recommended a local nanny agency. I found the agency to be fantastic as they match up an extensive list of criteria but again, it all comes at a hefty price.

Nannies tend to know other nannies and mention to each other when they are looking for a job or thinking about leaving their current position so ask any nannies you know to keep their ears to the ground and mention you are looking to their friends.

There are a number of websites where you can post adverts and where nannies post job-seeking adverts. You can search the database and e-mail the nannies you think may be suitable for you. You normally pay a fee to access these kind of website databases – but it is a lot less than an agency fee.

If you are going to find a nanny on your own, here are some things to remember:

- ❖ Check their qualifications
- ❖ Are they CRB checked?
- ❖ Is their insurance up-to-date?
- ❖ Do you want them to be Ofsted registered – if so, are you prepared to pay the fee if necessary?
- ❖ Check their references
- ❖ Do they know first aid?
- ❖ Anything else that is relevant or important to you

BECOMING AN EMPLOYER

Somewhat annoyingly, nannies fall outside the criteria of being self-employed, which means that you will need to become their employer. You have to register as an employer with Her Majesty's Revenue and Customs (HMRC). You have to provide your nanny with a payslip, pay their Pay As You Earn (PAYE) and National Insurance (NI) contributions.

There are companies that will take care of everything for you for a yearly subscription fee of around £200 - £300. They will send you your nanny's payslips once a month for you to give to your nanny, e-mail you when you need to pay your nanny's PAYE and NI contributions and tell you how much. They often have an in-house legal team and helplines should you have any problems or questions about holiday, sick pay or any other nanny related queries. Different providers offer slightly different services.

Providers include:

www.payefornannies.co.uk

www.nannypaye.co.uk

www.nannytax.co.uk

Should you wish to do it yourselves, check the HMRC website 'employers' page which should give you all the information you need. Alternatively you can call them and contrary to what you man think about the dreaded taxman, we found them to be very nice and helpful on the phone.

HMRC Contact details:

www.hmrc.gov.uk/employers 0845 714 3143

Offices are open from Monday to Friday, 8am to 8pm.

Interviewing Your Nanny

I honestly think that when it come to employing a nanny you will just *know* if they are the right fit for your family but if you have never interviewed anyone before here are a few things I would advise:

❖ Have a written list of any questions you know you want to ask. Check the list of 'Questions to Ask' on page 42, as a starting point.

❖ Have them come (maybe for their second interview when you are fairly certain you like them) when the children are still awake so you can see how they interact with your children and see what your children make of them.

❖ Have a very clear idea about what the job will entail and the things that you will expect them to do. The more information you can give them the better, as it will allow them to determine if it is the right job for them.

❖ Think about any additional assistance you will need (within reason, obviously). For example we asked our nanny when she was making dinner for the children, where possible, to cook extra so my husband could heat dinner up when he got in. Do some light grocery shopping when needed. Continue with the children's groups. Take them swimming once a week. We also include two evenings a month babysitting in their salary.

❖ Talk about the hours, start date, sick days, holiday days, time off over Christmas etc.

❖ If you know there are areas that are particularly challenging for your children (for me it was the fact that my son was a VERY fussy eater and every meal was a battle), tell them about it and ask how they would handle it.

The nanny needs to know that the job is going to work for them too so give them as much information about you and your family as possible. There is no point in them starting and then leaving a month later because the job isn't what they were expecting or you being unhappy because they aren't doing what you were expecting.

Be upfront and clear about what you want from the beginning and encourage them to do the same.

Your Nanny's Contract

If you decide to go ahead and hire a nanny you will need to provide them with a contract. If you have hired through an agency or are using a pay provider they should be able to help you write the contract or give you templates to use.

Here are some things to think about:

❖ **Holiday**

It is commonplace for your nanny to choose the dates for half their holiday time and for you to choose the other half. That way you can ask them to take holiday when you are away.

❖ **Babysitting**

We included two nights babysitting in our nanny's contract within her monthly salary and then specified how much we would pay her hourly if we would like her to babysit on top of that provision.

❖ **Driving and Mileage**

Whose car will the nanny drive? If it is her own, check her insurance and car documents are up-to-date. Agree how much you will pay for mileage, how it will be worked out and how often it will be paid. Our nanny kept a log for two weeks and then we worked out the average and gave her the cash each week, topping it up if she had longer drives for any reason.

❖ **Expenses**

We knew how much money our nanny was going to need for the week and would leave her cash for the week every Monday, but there are other options. You could give a pay-as-you-go card, a credit card or ask them to keep receipts and reimburse them at the end of the week.

FINAL THOUGHT

Of course we would love not to inflict serious illness on any children within our family – or anyone at all for that matter but that isn't the reality.

I remember when I was very upset after missing my daughter rolling over for the first time because I was at hospital and the nanny was looking after her. My husband said to me, "our daughter doesn't care if you were there to see her roll over or not, she cares if you are there for the rest of her life or not." This notion served me well throughout my treatment, reminding me that there is an end goal you are striving for and that is the important part of the process.

USEFUL CONTACTS

www.hmrc.gov.uk/employers
www.ofsted.gov.uk
www.payefornannies.co.uk
www.nannypaye.co.uk
www.nannytax.co.uk

Chapter Four

DOCTORS, HOSPITALS & TREATMENT

Courage doesn't always roar,
sometimes it's the quiet voice at the end of the day whispering,
'I will try again tomorrow.'
- Mary Ann Radmacher

CHOOSING YOUR HOSPITAL

Did you know that you can choose the NHS hospital you are treated in and the doctors who treat you? If not, neither did I until a surgeon told me. If so, you are already a step ahead of where I was, but either way, you can. You just need to ask your GP to refer you to the hospital of your choice. Even if your hospital of choice is in a different NHS Trust or in another county, you can choose that hospital.

There may be a few things you may want to consider:

❖ If a hospital or a particular doctor within a certain hospital specialises in the treatment of your specific type of cancer.

❖ Proximity to your home or more specifically, the travelling time.

   You will be going to hospital a lot for appointments, treatment, your operation, follow-up appointments, etc. so do think about this. Do you know someone who could drive you fairly regularly? Or how much would a taxi cost if needed?

   If you suffer from travel sickness then trust me, it's going to be worse after chemotherapy.

   Are there any other travel factors that are relevant to you?

❖ How easy it would be for your family and friends to visit? This may be very important if you are having long stays in hospital.

I chose a hospital a family member working at. It had a genetics programme, which was very important to me, given my family history. Plus, the surgeon had treated many women my age (which was unusual for my type of cancer). The hospital was a lot further than my local but I thought the positives outweighed the negatives, so I went for it.

If looking at various hospitals is something you are interested in doing, you can find information about hospitals online. The best website I found was, 'Dr Foster Heath'. You can search hospitals and specific consultants to match your illness and it gives a huge amount of information for each one.

www.drfosterhealth.co.uk

You can also check the NHS website where you can find reviews from users and staff. The website also has plenty of general information about the NHS. Everything from applying for medical exemption certificates (which you are entitled to when you have cancer so get yours now) to dentists so it is well worth a look.

www.nhs.uk

TOP TIP ABOUT DENTISTS

You can't have dental treatment whilst having chemotherapy. Go for a check up and have any necessary dental work done before you start your chemotherapy treatment.

HOW TO BE PREPARED FOR AN APPOINTMENT

At the beginning, fighting cancer is a bit of a snore-fest! Appointment after appointment, waiting room after waiting room. There are so many hours spent hanging around so:

❖ **Have a good book, magazine, game, fully charged phone, whatever can keep you distracted for long periods of time.** You don't need me to tell you that doctors aren't great at running on time, so you might as well make it pass more pleasantly.

❖ **Have your appointment card or letter with you.** It is so much easier for everyone, especially the receptionist. Having said that, I used to forget mine all the time and they always found me on the system so don't panic if you forget, but still, it does make life easier.

❖ **Think about your appointment before going, write down any questions** that you can think of and take them with you because in the moment you may get distracted by something they say and forget, then remember the minute you walk out of the room. It happens to me all the time and is so annoying.

❖ **Don't let the doctor rush you.** If you have a question, however small, ask it. Remember – that's the point of the appointment!

❖ **Take your notes.** There can be a lack of communication between hospital departments who do not seem to handover your notes to each other. You will get asked the same questions over and over again, especially at the beginning. The main questions being about your medical history and current conditions.

You can ask your GP for a print out of your medical history and list of medications you are on so that you can take a copy with you. Save repeating yourself.

5 TOP TIPS FOR HAVING A SCAN

I have had quite a few scans over the years and I have learnt a few things that are well worth remembering when going for a scan.

❖ Unless you are rather partial to the 'property of the NHS, do not remove' printed gown, don't wear anything with metal on. By that I mean zips, buttons and wires. As long as you have no metal you can normally keep your clothes on and don't have to change into a hospital gown.
The no metal rule includes underwire bras.

❖ If the hospital send you a drink to drink before your scan, there is no positive way to spin it, the drink they send you tastes disgusting! I have tried it with every flavor cordial and I can confirm that blackcurrant masks the taste the best. Don't hold back when adding cordial. This isn't lightly flavoring water, it's making something disgusting drinkable so my advice, go for it!

❖ A chaser. Unfortunately I don't mean anything to exciting, but with some of the scans you can eat and drink so I like to follow it straight up with a drink I like the taste of to 'cleanse my pallet.' Personally I found Sprite the best chaser, gives a nice clean taste. **Check if this is OK with the type of scan you are having. With some, such as a PET scan, you cannot eat or drink before.**

❖ Allow a fair bit of time either side of your appointment. As well as needing you to be there early, the nurses will usually ask you to stay for fifteen minutes or so afterwards to make sure you are feeling OK after your scan.

❖ Try not to panic. Easy to say I know but the scan operators are only on the other side of the glass and can clearly see and hear you. You are in safe hands, so do not worry.

HAVING CHEMOTHERAPY

Chemotherapy is a medication used to treat cancer that is traditionally given intravenously through a drip. Some types of chemotherapy are now available in a tablet form, or you may be given, what I had, which is a combination of both. Chemotherapy is carried around your body through the blood stream so that it can try and break down cancerous cells anywhere in the body.

There are *so* many types of chemotherapy. All of which come with different side effects. Your oncologist should give you information about common side effects associated with your type of chemotherapy. However, in my experience, the doctors didn't want to give me too much information about possible side effects. It's like the self-fulfilling prophecy: if someone says you will get a headache, suddenly, you have a headache. Instead they don't say anything and wait to see what side effects you experience. I understand the theory but I would have appreciated some warning on what was to come and knowing what would be considered a 'normal' reaction and what would be considered 'extreme'.

If your doctor has not given you as much information as you would like, you should be able to find out through the MacMillan or Cancer Research UK websites.

www.cancerresearchuk.org

www.macmillan.org.uk

TOP TIP

Keep a daily diary of how you are feeling physically and emotionally, noting any changes from one day to the next.

When you are having chemotherapy or radiotherapy you will meet with a doctor regularly to assess how you are getting on. It is amazing how much you can forget about how you feel straight after chemotherapy when you next see your oncologist a few weeks later.

Keep an eye on levels of nausea, how many times you are sick, any pain or discomfort (and if so, where), energy levels, and your mood. It will give you and your oncologist a clear idea of how your treatment is affecting you at different points.

What to Expect During Chemotherapy

A *lot* of hanging around! You will probably have a blood test and be weighed either that morning or the day before you have chemotherapy, as the amount of chemotherapy you are given is worked out on your weight, and the blood tests ensures your body is strong enough to have chemotherapy.

Treatment is given in a chemotherapy suite, which will comprise of comfy chairs and sometimes beds where you will sit or lie whilst having treatment.

> ### JUST SO YOU KNOW
> *You will need the toilet a lot during your chemotherapy session as the medication is given in large amounts of fluid, but fear not, there is usually a toilet in the chemo suite. The nurses can unplug your IV machine so don't feel like you are trapped to staying where you are, just ask one of the nurses.*

What to Take to Chemotherapy

❖ **Something to read, watch or play.** Generally you will be in hospital for hours. I would find about halfway through my treatment my concentration would evaporate, so I couldn't do much. I found weekly magazines good because its light entertainment delivered in bite-size chunks.

❖ **A microwaveable lavender pillow** – They usually have these in chemotherapy suites; so don't worry if you don't have one.

❖ **Mints** to keep your mouth fresh.

❖ **Take a scarf, gloves and hat to wear on your way home**. Your senses will be seriously over sensitised after treatment. A blanket in the car is also quite nice. I was always exhausted after my treatment so used to get really comfy in the car and just chill.

Straight After Chemotherapy

You may not be well enough to drive after chemotherapy, so have someone collect you or put arrangements in place for getting home, prior to your chemotherapy appointment. Some hospitals offer a 'collect and drop off' service, so speak with the receptionists what your hospital can offer.

THE BENEFITS OF A PICC LINE

A PICC (peripherally inserted central catheter) line is a small tube that is inserted into a vein in your upper arm and threads through the vein to just above your heart.

Unsurprisingly, your veins do not like chemotherapy so they constrict to try and stop it getting in to your system, which can actually be quite painful. The warmth from the lavender pillows helps the veins to release which helps to alleviate the pain. Some women I met during chemotherapy found that the pillows worked brilliantly, whereas for me it didn't and I would still be in great discomfort.

However, the PICC line eliminates the discomfort completely, delivering the chemotherapy straight to the heart, skipping the veins completely. It depends how much discomfort you are experiencing whilst receiving chemotherapy as to whether you will want one.

I refused a PICC line for ages after the nurses suggested it to me. I didn't want yet another procedure to have it fitted and I wasn't entirely sure about the whole idea of having a line thread through my vein.

If I'm honest it was uncomfortable having it fitted and it took a little while. It did feel strange at first but quickly I couldn't feel it at all. However, what really matters is that it revolutionised having chemotherapy for me, making it a thousand times easier. I honestly wish I had got one fitted immediately. Given how unpleasant chemotherapy is, anything that can make it easier is, in my mind, well worth it.

If you are interested in having a PICC line fitted, ask your oncologist or oncological nurse.

HAVING RADIOTHERAPY

Radiotherapy is literally a radiation ray or beam that is concentrated on the sight of your cancer. During a radiotherapy treatment, you lie on a bed and a radioactive beam is targeted towards the specific area affected by cancer by a large x-ray type machine. Essentially, the radioactive beam blasts the cancerous cells into submission! It's not too dissimilar to having an x-ray and you shouldn't feel anything whilst actually having the treatment. Radiotherapy is usually given daily over a period; in my case it was every day for six weeks (apart from weekends, hospitals tend not to fight cancer on the weekend – except in extreme cases).

Your CT or MRI scan will be used to determine exactly where radiologists will aim the machine, then you are given tiny tattoos (I literally mean a dot, smaller than a freckle, that you will never be able to find afterwards) so that they are able to aim the radiotherapy beam to the exact same place every time.

There will inevitably be some healthy tissue damaged by radiotherapy. The use of scans and tattoos will ensure the damage is minimal, however burning, similar to sunburn, should be expected.

What to Take to Radiotherapy

❖ Book, magazine, tablet etc. for the waiting.
❖ The rooms are kept very cool to stop the machines overheating so keep the parts of your body that aren't exposed well covered.

After Your Treatment

Radiotherapy can burn the skin quite badly. In my case it was very uncomfortable as it burnt my undercarriage making it very difficult to use the toilet. I know a lady who had breast cancer and couldn't wear a bra as it rubbed on the burnt skin that she described as being 'like a sunburn.'

Take particular care of your skin during this time. Keep burnt skin out of the hot sunshine and avoid products that dry the skin.

YOUR HOSPITAL STAY

I don't think staying in hospital conjures up happy thoughts for anyone but it will probably be a necessary part of your cancer treatment, so let's try and make it as pleasant as possible.

How to Pack for a Hospital Stay

I knew I was going to be in hospital for at least ten days following my surgery. I took in so many books, my laptop and lists of little jobs I could do from my hospital bed. I hadn't truly accounted for just how crap I was going to feel and I didn't end up doing any of that! Seeing loved ones and sleeping was about all I was good for.

Here is a list of the things I could not have lived without or that I wished I'd had:

- ❖ Dressing gown
- ❖ Nightie – I would go for a nightie over pyjamas, as you will probably have a catheter fitted after the operation meaning you wouldn't be able to wear pyjama bottoms initially anyway.
- ❖ Mobile phone and charger
- ❖ Ear plugs
- ❖ Wet wipes
- ❖ Hand gel for use before meals and for any visitors
- ❖ Some change for when those lovely ladies and

gentlemen come round with a trolley full of chocolate (but not to much money as there is never anywhere you keep things completely safe).

TOP TIP

Put pictures of your loved ones and little (inexpensive) mementos from home all around your bed.

The day after my operation my husband brought in drawings our children had done for me, 'get well' cards and a small figurine from my bedside table at home and set them up around my bed.

It made such a difference when I was feeling horrible to have these lovely things to look at and it made the hospital feel as homely as is possible when you are wearing a gown with 'hospital property do not remove' written all over it – seriously, who is *ever* going to steal that gown?

I would strongly urge anyone who is going into hospital to do this, even if you are only going to be in hospital for a couple of days.

DAY 3 & DAY 10 HOSPITAL BLUES

On the third day of my hospital stay, I was feeling so low that I burst into tears when my surgeon came in and asked me that dreaded question when you are feeling emotional – 'How are you?' Cue serious amounts of tears!

Thankfully, she told me this was normal and is known as the 'day three blues'. No one really knows why you get the 'day three blues' but it is thought to be a combination of relief that the surgery is over and that you survived it, the reality of physical changes to your body, being stuck in hospital and a strong side effect to the anaesthetic as it starts to leave your body. With such an awful combination of mixed emotional feelings and physical symptoms, it's no wonder that the 'day three blues' is a real thing!

My advice would be, know that it is par for the course and don't let it worry you. You are experiencing something that is completely natural and expected but know that, it will pass. Let yourself go through the emotion the best you can and if you need to cry... have a good cry damn it! Let it out, and then remember how amazing you are for going through another stage of cancer treatment.

If You Are Not Happy With Your Hospital

Most hospitals have a Patient Liaison Service, commonly known as PALS, with whom you or a relative can speak with about any concerns in regards to the hospital, doctors or treatment. You can also make an official complaint to PALS.

If your hospital doesn't have PALS, check

www.pals.nhs.uk to find the nearest one and they will be able to help you.

COMING HOME AFTER YOUR HOSPITAL STAY

Your experience of surgery and staying in hospital is over and you are finally home – yay! I honestly thought that when I got home, everything would be fine but it didn't work out quite like that. I hadn't planned for quite such a long recovery.

Visitors

Once you get home, you may have the world and their wife wanting to visit. Suddenly the visiting hours that were once annoyingly restricting and the nurse, who firmly kicked everyone out, are missed, as guests stay longer than you would like. People who aren't ill just don't realise how much lying down and talking to someone can take out of you – it's exhausting – seriously!

I used to find that when I was worn out, I needed to take more painkillers as my whole body would ache with tiredness and feel very uncomfortable. It's hardly surprising, you are still convalescing, your body is trying to heal and you need to let it, which means a huge amount of proper, uninterrupted, rest. Do let visitors know if it is getting too much!

> ## TOP TIP
>
> *I found it useful when making an arrangement to say, "I am trying to keep visits to thirty-minutes (or whatever length of time you are comfortable with) otherwise it's too much for me". That way, people come with an expectation of when to leave. I also didn't feel so rude if I had to remind a visitor of the time.*
>
> *When my mother was ill, my sister or I used to knock on the door after thirty-minutes and remind mum that she needed to sleep which was also a subtle way of reminding visitors their time was up, it worked really well. So if you don't feel comfortable reminding visitors to leave, ask someone else in the house to do it for you.*

Now is a great time to call in all those "Can I do anything to help?" offers. Ask visitors to bring healthy meals so you don't have to cook, do the hovering whilst they are there, pick up some milk on their way... Whatever it is that you need and is going to make your life easier.

Just think, when your cancer is gone, you won't have any leverage to ask people to help you do this stuff, so make the most of it now!

Boudoir Sanctuary

If you are spending time recovering after your operation and therefore in bed, you want to try and make your bedroom as a tranquil, heavenly place that you want to be in. This means:

❖ Try to keep your room clean and tidy.
❖ Open a window at least once a day, even if it is only for a few minutes, to keep the fresh air circulating.
❖ Get someone to change your sheets every few days. Decadent yes, but trust me, you will feel so much better for it.
❖ Flowers always brighten a room!
❖ Display photo's that will keep you uplifted, inspired and remind you what you are fighting for.

TOP TIP FROM MY WARD NURSE

This was the best piece of advice I was given by a nurse on my ward when I was leaving hospital…

Every morning, regardless of how tired you are or how badly you've slept, get up, have a wash and get dressed. Even if it is only into a tracksuit and you get straight back into bed afterwards and go to sleep (which I often did), still get up, washed and dressed. In the evening, get ready for bed and into your pyjamas.

Mentally, this will give you a distinction between night and day, which can be invaluable physically and especially mentally when you are spending a lot of time in bed. Otherwise, you can end up staying in bed, in your pj's, not changing the sheets – all of which can make you feel down and you do not want that!

Getting Out the House

As much as you may not feel like it, believe me when I say, fresh air can be the best medicine. Getting out and about gets the blood circulating, oxygen filling your cells and after being cooped up in a hospital, it's just wonderful, and you will feel so much better for it.

Just a small walk to the nearest lamppost and back will be fine at first, and then build a little more every day. Have a little celebration party when you make it to the end of the street.

If you really don't feel well enough to walk anywhere, maybe think about borrowing a wheelchair? You can 'borrow' one from the British Red Cross, just call your local centre. They loan wheelchairs for four weeks at a time. You will still get the benefit from bring outside, seeing some nature and getting fresh air. There are local British Red Cross centres throughout the UK. Check their website to find the closest one to you. www.redcross.org.uk

MOST IMPORTANTLY

As I have said time and time again, be kind to yourself. Recovery is a process that takes time and it may feel like an annoyingly long process but every day is a step in the right direction.

You have just got through something major so be extra kind and loving to your amazing self!

USEFUL CONTACTS

www.nhs.uk
www.drfosterhealth.co.uk
www.pals.nhs.uk
www.redcross.org.uk
www.cancerresearchuk.org
www.macmillan.org.uk

Chapter Five

THE EMOTIONAL ROLLERCOASTER

The more I think of it,
the more I realise there are no answers.
Life is to be lived.
- Marilyn Monroe

Going through cancer, you can often feel like you are fighting an emotional battle as well as a physical one. In some ways the emotional side is the hardest part of cancer.

You have just crashed into a frightening, unrelenting face-off with your own mortality, and what is causing this horrendous condition? Your own body! Your body has waged war on itself and your sanity can feel like the prize it is fighting over. You are coping with being ill, loved ones, treatment, surgery, let alone attempting to live your normal life and all that it brings.

THE MANY EMOTIONS OF CANCER

When you have cancer, some of the emotions you experience are emotions everyone expects you to have – feelings like anger, sorrow, fear and a general feeling of being over-whelmed or worn-out with it all. But there are so many other emotions you don't hear about as much.

I was speaking with a friend, who has also had cancer about all the unexpected emotions we had felt and it turned out they were the same, it suddenly seemed strange that we had never spoken about it before. I hope that in talking about these emotions you will know that if you are feeling them too, you are not alone.

Relief

I felt a certain amount of relief when I was diagnosed. This may sound strange but I had known that something was wrong for sometime so to know that I wasn't going crazy or not eating enough fiber (as the GP kept saying) was a strange sort of relief. At least now we knew what it was, we could start trying to deal with it.

Guilt

This is a big one. And many other Cancer Superstars I know say the same. There are so many facets to the guilt as well.

Guilt that you are inflicting this illness on others. Guilt if certain family members or friends are coping very well. Guilt that you are doing better than the person sitting next to you having chemotherapy. Guilt over getting the all clear when someone else didn't. Guilt over not being around for your kids as much as you should have been. Guilt over eating red meat or drinking bottled water (or whatever the latest, 'this will give you cancer' is) that could have possibly brought you to having the disease. Guilt over not acknowledging just how bad it was when someone else was going through cancer before you because you didn't realise *just* how much they would be going through. Guilt, guilt, guilt, guilt, guilt!

Whenever you mention this to anyone who hasn't had cancer, again they look at you like you are mad. To be fair, it does sound mad. None of those things are your fault and thinking about it logically, by definition you should only feel guilty if you have done something wrong.

But that's the amazing thing about emotions, they can be completely irrational and yet retain their strength and conviction over the person who is feeling them.

Not The Right Emotion

Sometimes you may not have the emotion or reaction that others expect you to have. For me it was it was the 'why me' emotion. I never felt this. People would say 'you must be thinking, why me' and when I said I no I didn't, people would look at me like I was crazy… or lying! I did feel 'why now' and thought the timing was unfair given that I had a tiny baby and toddler when I was diagnosed but never why me.

My friend felt like she had to apologies for not being

emotional enough and crying all the time. I think people often think I'm strange that I am able to talk about it so matter-of-factly and not break down every time. I don't know why this is. Just because I'm feeling strong at that moment, doesn't mean I'm not going to break down later that day / weekend / whenever. No one can sustain that level of heightened emotion with a constant outpouring of feelings. It doesn't mean you're not feeling it, but people sometimes find that hard to understand when they can't *see* you feeling it.

My two-year-old only has room for one emotion at a time so can go from a screaming fit to laughing in a nano-second but adults and especially one's who have cancer don't act like that. The number of conflicting emotions that you can be feeling at anyone time when you have cancer is cataclysmic and enough to give you a serious headache. There can be so many different emotions in your heart at any one time.

REMEMBER

There are no right or wrong emotions. Everyone is going to handle it differently depending on his or her constitution and circumstances. Whatever you are feeling is completely normal.

THE PROVERBIAL EMOTIONAL ROLLERCOASTER

I once received a message from a lady praising my positive attitude to having cancer. This lady also went on to say that her son had cancer and that he was in a very negative place. She said that she had tried encouraging him to read my blog, to gain a different perspective but said that he wasn't interested, that he was so fearful for the future and she asked if I ever felt like that?

I wrote back saying **'*YES!*'**

Her question made me think about how important it is to discuss the lowest lows that you go through when dealing with cancer.

In writing this book, I wanted to write something inspirational and positive, but not just to try and convince everyone that it is a plain sailing, positive inducing experience. I certainly do not want anyone to feel that to beat cancer you must think positively or you will be condemning yourself to death penalty for not doing so. I have a wonderful friend who stayed positive throughout her whole treatment. She told me that she never allowed herself to think the worst. She felt that remaining positive was integral to getting better and never allowed negativity to creep into her thoughts.

I did not feel like this!

There were days when I felt utterly lost in the darkest depths of an abyss. Like one of those little sea-creatures that lives in a place so dark its blind and has no idea which way is up or down, that was me. There were times when all I wanted to do was hide away. Treatment and bed - that was it for me. At some points that was all I was physically able to do but at other points, it was a very useful excuse. As I started to recognise this pattern, I tried to keep plans, or even invite my dad or sister round when I felt low and didn't want to see anyone, which did help.

> ### TOP TIP
> *When you are feeling low, try not to shut yourself away. You are more likely to feel better for seeing someone or doing something rather than being locked away on your own.*

Lowest of the Low

Your lowest moments may not be when you would expect. I found the lead up to my twelve-hour operation mind-crushingly hard. I was petrified that I would go to sleep and never wake up. I was so scared, I couldn't even discuss my fears with anyone. In the end I had to push myself to tell one of my closest friends how scared I was because I wanted her to be able to pass on messages to my husband and children should my worst fear become reality. I don't think anyone can fully understand the physical internal pain caused by the fear I experienced in the weeks leading up to my operation.

My other 'lowest of the low' actually came towards the end of my treatment, which might sound strange – it certainly did to those around me. I reached a point where I couldn't fight anymore. I was so physically and mentally tired, I didn't have any more fight left in me. People kept saying 'Why? You're so close to the end.' Yet all I could think was 'I can't have another three-months of chemotherapy.' I had reached a point where I would rather give up completely than even think about keeping going.

I spoke to my oncology nurse about it and she was very understanding. I think that sometimes as cancer sufferers we can assume our reactions are unique, but clearly nurses see ranges of emotions all the time. She advised antidepressants to give me the boost that I needed to get me through the last few months of treatment.

Previously I had been quite 'anti' anti-depressants but at that point, I was on so many tablets counteracting side effects from the cancer and treatment that I figured 'what's one more tablet a day?' Plus I acknowledged that I needed extra help. The antidepressants did help and got me through the end of my treatment. I'm not suggesting antidepressants are the answer for everyone, but for me they were and still are very effective. If you are also not keen on the thought of anti-depressants, it may be worth staying open-minded about the various options that are available to you.

I must admit that I have felt quite emotional writing these pages of the book, remembering the feeling of that long dormant fear in the pit of my stomach. But if you feel this way, or have a loved one who does, just know that it is inevitably part of the process.

I think the reason that I am able to speak about cancer so positively now is because I am cancer free. People generally (myself definitely) have an incredible knack for looking back on experiences and extracting meaning and positivity from them. That doesn't mean that the 'meaning' was obvious at the time. Or even necessarily there. I have turned out fine! In every way, I think my life is even better than before. I have done things I wanted to do my whole life but never had the guts to do before. Ironic as it was my guts that had cancer and are now gone – a little bit of 'cancer humor' there.

REMEMBER

Take everyday as it comes. One day can vary so much to the next, sometimes you just have to ride out the bad days and enjoy the good ones. Most importantly you have to be kind to yourself and remember every feeling you are feeling, no matter how extreme, is part of your process.

A BAD DAY

You will have bad days. It is an unfortunate inevitability you just have to accept – generally in life, but *particularly* during cancer. I would swing between thinking 'I can totally do this' to 'I give up, just let me die.' Sounds dramatic now but that truly was how I felt at certain moments.

It's fair to say that these moments often coincided with a huge dose of chemotherapy or a terrible night's sleep due to the discomfort caused by radiotherapy. I soon learnt to just accept bad days as part of the treatment process. I would do what I could to alleviate these feelings and say to myself over and over again (as some sort of calming mantra), 'this too shall pass'.

This Too Shall Pass

If there is one thing I have learnt over the last couple of years of cancer treatment, the aftershock, child rearing and life in general, it is that these feelings do pass, life will go on and in another day (or another hour in some cases) things will become easier. In essence – *this too shall pass.*

The fantastic thing I have found by thinking 'this too shall pass' when things are rough, is that it stops me falling into too much of a downward spiral. It reminds me to try and accept my emotions for what they are. Sometimes tricky, sometimes difficult but I try to let them wash over me, move on and help myself where I can.

I remember one instance when I was writing on my blog about an awful day I was having. I had hay fever so bad it was making my head foggy and my eyes and nose would not stop running. My children were doing everything they know they shouldn't and completely ignoring me when I tried to retain some semblance of control. Worst of all, I had a horrendous leak from my colostomy bag. Had I been out and about, I would have classed it as one of the most embarrassing experiences of my life. Thankfully I was at home so I was able to sort myself out discreetly.

There are days when I handle everything that has happened to me and my toddlers terrible two's with (what I hope is) a positive grace, but there are other days when its hard and I wish I didn't have to deal with any of it. This was one of those days.

REMEMBER

Negative emotions are a part of life and an inability to talk about them can leave people feeling isolated and like they are the only one. So here you are, confirmation that if you are having bad day then you are not alone.

So this day when I was feeling at the end of my tether, began with a trip to Boots to buy a million Loperamide's (which helps to take water out of the colon and should stop another leak) and taking the children to an indoor soft play center to burn off some hyperactivity and I could sit and write, which I find deeply therapeutic. Of course, in no time at all the worst had passed and my spirits lifted. But I also know this positivity will also pass. I will feel blue again, however when it does I will be able to think to myself again, *this too shall pass.*

What Can I Do on a Bad Day?

❖ **Take some Rescue Remedy**

They also do a Rescue Remedy Night Time, designed to help you sleep which I found fabulous.

❖ **Talk to someone**

Get a friend or family member round to talk about things or talk about something completely different if you prefer.

❖ **Go for a walk**

Walking is proven to lift someone's mood. The combination of fresh air and gentle exercise is a winner every time, especially if you are spending time cooped up in doors.

❖ **Gardening**

Even if you aren't much of a gardener, again it's about getting outside and gentle movement.

❖ **Get back to nature**

There is something very healing about nature as well. I can't explain it, but do try and get out in nature as much as possible, even if it is just sitting in a garden.

❖ **Counselling or**
Cognitive Behavioural Therapy

Either may be a good idea (see more on both below), especially if your bad days are becoming more common than not, talking therapy can be very effective.

DEPRESSION

Towards the end of my treatment and, interestingly, after I got the all clear, I had to admit that these 'bad days' weren't just days anymore. They were weeks that were turning into months. Not good! I had to recognise that I was depressed.

How can you tell the difference bad days and depression? You can't 'shake off' depression. It is with you all the time and you, or your loved ones, will probably be able to tell when you are feeling depressed.

Some of the things to look out for include:

- ❖ Feeling very negative about yourself
- ❖ Not feeling in control of your emotions or feelings
- ❖ Feeling unable to face the world or other people
- ❖ Not wanting to leave the house
- ❖ Feeling detached from your own life
- ❖ Wanting to harm yourself in any way
- ❖ If you have suffered with depression before, recognising similar symptoms.

Reactive or Chemical?

Depression is sometimes split into two categories, reactive or chemical.

As you may expect, reactive is called so because it is a reaction to an extreme circumstance – like having cancer, but it could also be through grief or a particularly upsetting time.

Chemical depression is where the levels of serotonin in the brain have fallen beneath their normal levels after a continuous period of dealing with negative situations in your life – like having cancer, which makes you feel depressed.

WHAT CAN I DO?

Whether you are having a bad day or think you may have depression, the first thing to do is speak to someone involved in your treatment.

If you are currently having chemotherapy or radiotherapy you should be meeting with a doctor regularly. Make sure you tell them about any emotional changes or concerns as well as the physical effects. The good thing about seeing someone in oncology is that they will be aware of all the medication you are currently on and what would work sympathetically. If you are not currently in cancer treatment or having regular check-ups you should still be able to speak to someone in your dedicated team.

If you have a good GP, you could speak with them and in fact your oncology team may advise going directly to your GP. A lot of practices now offer counselling and Cognitive Behavioural Therapy (known as CBT), as well as anti-depressants and alternative prescribed medication.

Your local cancer centre (mentioned in chapter 2, Friends, Family and Home) will most likely also offer a form of talking therapy. The added benefit is that their therapists will specialise in working with people with cancer, and all the specific challenges that brings.

COUNSELLING

One of the most common 'talking therapies' is counselling. It involves just that – talking, and lots of it. The counsellor will be skilled in drawing concerns out of you, encouraging you to get to the root of what is bothering you so you can discuss it in a non-judgemental, safe place.

I had counselling and remember walking in the room thinking 'what on earth I am going to say to this woman… for an hour!' One moment I was shifting awkwardly in my seat but the next moment I was chatting away, unable to believe it when my time was up. All sorts just came flooding out. The counsellor I saw was so wonderful. As well as listening, she was able to offer me insights into how I was feeling, which helped me feel more in control of my emotions.

Where to Find a Counsellor
* Through your oncological team or GP
* At your local cancer centre
* The an accredited society such as
  o British Association for Counselling and Psychotherapy (BACP) www.bacp.co.uk
  o National Counselling Society www.nationalcounsellingsociety.org

COGNITIVE BEHVIOURAL THERAPY

This is fast becoming a go-to for doctors when prescribing someone a talking therapy. Again you are given an opportunity to talk about how you are feeling or anything that is concerning you. The difference is that in CBT you are taught techniques to help you look at things in a different way and should those feelings or concerns arise again, you are better equipped to deal with them or have a different way of looking at things.

For example, a fear of mine was that the cancer would come back and I would die from cancer before I was fifty like my mothers did. The counsellor asked about my father's health – which is relatively impeccable - and reminded me that I carry his DNA too.

There are a number of techniques they can use. Your therapist will decide which is best suited to your individual situation.

Where to Find a Cognitive Behavioural Therapist
❖ Through your oncological team or GP
❖ At your local cancer centre
❖ The an accredited society such as
      ○ British Association for Behavioural and Cognitive Psychotherapies (BABCP) www.babcp.com
      ○ National Association of Cognitive Behavioural Therapists (NACBT) www.nacbt.org

ANTI-DEPRESSANTS

Anti-depressants are a prescribed medication that help to balance chemicals and hormones in the brain and body to keep your emotions on an even keel.

Prior to having cancer, I was not a fan of anti-depressants. I always felt you should treat the cause. You should think about why you are depressed and deal with that. Now I have been depressed I found myself eating my words and I now appreciate that it's not always that straightforward. Towards the end of my last bout of chemotherapy I was really starting to feel like I just couldn't go on. It was more than feeling 'a bit low' or having a 'bad day' because everyone has down days from time-to-time. This was less like a 'bad day' and more like 'I'm calling time on this.'

As I said in the 'Lowest of the Low,' (pages 75 – 77) I spoke to my oncological nurse to let her know that I couldn't do it anymore. She listened and helped put things back in perspective. She also suggested putting me on a low dose of anti-depressants to take the edge off and get me through to the end of my treatment. Logically I knew finishing my treatment had to be done. At this point I was struggling so much emotionally, I would have cut my right-arm off to feel better, taking a tiny pill seemed like a much easier and less-dramatic solution. It worked, it took the edge off and I got through the end of the treatment. It did take a little while to get the type of anti-depressant and levels correct but once we did, every thing felt *so* much easier.

If you have Chemical Depression anti-depressants

can help to bring the level of serotonin back up to a normal level, giving you that boost you will need to deal with everything else you are going through.

FINDING OUT MORE

Depression, bad days and the whole emotional side of cancer can be a large area to think about so as I said before, if you are unsure, concerned or just need to talk to someone, **do speak with a member of your oncology team or your GP.** For further information on mental health, you can check the MIND website.

USEFUL CONTACTS

www.cancerresearchuk.org
www.macmillan.org.uk
www.mind.org.uk
www.babcp.com
www.nacbt.org
www.bacp.co.uk
www.nationalcounsellingsociety.org

Chapter Six

STAYING SOCIAL WHEN STAYING IN

The happiest people do not have the best of everything,
they make the best of everything.
- Unknown

You may feel like cancer is robbing you of many things, including your social life. It can make you feel quite low when people are heading out and you aren't feeling well enough to join in. I often found the days that I wanted to see people the least ended up being the days I benefited from seeing people the most.

Don't let not being able to go out stop you seeing loved one's. Get your friends round and get involved with some of these fun, at home, ideas.

THROW A PAMPER PARTY

Personally I love evenings spent at home with girlfriends and you can turn these evenings into a fun but super relaxing spa time, enjoying a pamper evening.

In a former life I was a spa therapist and I have listed all the wonderful parts of spa therapy that can do at home below to make you evening even more fabulous!

You could prepare some gorgeous healthy snacks or ask everyone to bring something to save you the hassle of doing anything. For drinks, how about herbal tea, water or one of the fabulous juice recipes from the diet section? Who am I kidding, wine!

You could all truly get into the spirit of a spa event and bring dressing gowns, hairbands and face cloths. Put on some relaxing music and try some of these ideas:

How to Give the Perfect Facial

- ❖ **Cleanse** - Smooth a lovely cleanser all over the face and neck, in a gentle sweeping movement. Massage the cleaner into the skin in small circular motions. Be careful not to pull the skin and don't get to close to the eyes. Wipe the cleanser off your face with a damp face cloth or cotton wool.

- ❖ **Cleanse again** - The first cleanse will get rid of all the surface rubbish and make-up, the second is to work a little deeper. Exactly the same as before but let the massage go on for slightly longer, making sure you get into every part of the face – don't go to close to the eyes.

❖ **Tone** - You don't have to buy fancy toners. Rose Water (for normal or dry skin) or Lavender Water (for combination and oily skin) work just as well. Apply to clean, dry cotton wool and wipe over the whole face, getting rid of any left over cleanser or dirt residue.

❖ **Exfoliate** - With your own face scrub or one of the 'make you own' combinations listed below. Apply to the face and neck, again avoiding the eyes. Massage the exfoliator in with small circular movements. Wash off with warm water.

❖ **Steam** - This is an optional step and depends slightly on your skin type. I wouldn't advise it if you skin is very sensitive.

Boil a kettle, pour the water into a large bowl and lean over the bowl, with a towel draped over you and the bowl to catch all the steam for five minutes. The steam will open pores, allowing for a deep clean. Dab skin dry afterwards with a clean tissue or towel.

❖ **Mask** - Apply one of the super easy mask recipes listed below over the face, pop some cucumber over your eyes, sit back and relax. After five or ten minutes, wash off with warm water.

❖ **Treatment oil** - Ladies are often afraid of putting oils on their face, thinking it will make them look greasy, it's a common misconception as treatment oil's can be of great benefit.

TOP TIP

If your skin does appear greasy then you may be using too much oil. You only need a tiny drop.

The benefit of oil is that the molecules are so much smaller than a cream so they can sink deeper into the skin.

If you do use too much oil you can remove the excess by placing a tissue over the skin and letting it absorb the excess.

Don't rub the excess oil off, just dab.

❖ **Moisturise** - As well as keeping your skin soft, your mask acts as a barrier to the world and all its pollutants so it's worth having a good moisturiser. Dab a small amount over the face and neck, right down to your collarbone. Massage your moisturiser in with soothing, sweeping, upward movements. Again you can use a tissue to remove any excess.

Et voila! Beautiful, clean and nourished complexion.

How to Make A Face Mask

All Skin Types:	Mix together a tablespoon of honey, 3 tablespoons of yogurt and a few drops of lemon.
Cleansing Mask:	Smear honey on to damp skin.
Normal / Dry Skin:	Crush a banana with a fork and smooth on your face and neck.
Oily Skin:	Crush six strawberries with a fork and smooth on you face and neck.
Mature Skin:	Mix 1 avocado, 1 teaspoon of clear honey, 1 teaspoon of lemon juice and 1 teaspoon of plain yogurt, mashing it all together with a fork. Leave in the fridge for thirty minutes. Smooth over your skin.

How to Make an Exfoliator

- ❖ Pour half a cup of Coconut Oil (or you could use Olive, Almond or Grapeseed Oil) into a bowl
- ❖ Add 2 tablespoons of sugar.
- ❖ Squeeze in some lemon juice
- ❖ Mix together. Rubbing into the skin gently using small circular motions.

How to Make a Face Treatment Oil

Almond oil makes a great base product as it is full of nourishing vitamins and minerals and is easily absorbed by the skin.

Geranium is an excellent essential oil for all skin types and it facilitates cell turnover, which encourages new, radiant skin.

Lavender essential oil is fantastic for all skin types, balancing the skin and gives your skin whatever it needs so it is always a good idea!

- ❖ Quarter cup of Almond Oil
- ❖ Add 3 drops of Geranium and 3 drops of Lavender essential oils.
- ❖ Mix well.

If you have any left over (or wish to make extra), it is always best to store oils in dark glass jars, but remember it wont last for too long. I often buy dark glass bottles with pipettes making it easier to apply.

Manicures and Pedicures

- ❖ Fill a washing up bowl for your feet, dessert bowl for your hands, with warm water and a few drops of your favorite bubble bath.
- ❖ Soak your hands or feet for five minutes.
- ❖ Give your hands or feet a massage with oil or body lotion to ease out all the aches and pains or, even better, see if someone else will do it.

> *TOP MANUCIRE AND PEDICURE TIP*
>
> *If you are going to paint your nails afterwards, make sure that you wipe your nails with nail varnish remover first, to remove any oil or lotion otherwise the paint wont go on smoothly or grip to the nails properly.*

COME DINE WITH ME

You must have seen the show? The one where four strangers (generally strange) take it in turns to host dinner for each other at their homes over the course of a week and the best host wins £1000? Well I'm not quite suggesting that you invite strangers into your home, or give anyone a £1000 but how about having three or four friends cook you dinner?

How it Works

The challenge is for each person to serve a three-course meal and the guests, you included, secretly mark the chef, out of ten, on the success of the evening. The next person hosts dinner and so on. Once everyone has hosted an evening the scores are revealed and someone is announced the WINNER!

The meals don't have to be done in a week. I would probably recommend a couple of weeks between each one but really it comes down to how you are feeling and how tired you get.

You can put all kinds of parameters on the evenings to make them suit you better.

- ❖ You could make part of the challenge that they have to come to your house and make the meal and clear up afterwards so you don't have to go anywhere or do anything.
- ❖ Make cost part of the challenge, saying that each chef is only allowed to spend a certain amount on ingredients.
- ❖ Rather than all voting you can be the 'Queen Judge' and decide the winner!

The Short Version

If you don't want to spread it over a few evenings you could do it in one evening with three friends. One friend does the starter, one does the main and one does the dessert. All have dinner together and score each other's dishes. Simple.

The Prize

A few ideas... Obviously your friends will have been spending money on ingredients so you could spend that money on a gift voucher for the winner. The chefs could all chip in a couple of quid to enter so the winner wins the kitty. The knowledge that they are the best cook is clearly the best prize!

FILM CLUB

My husband and I became addicted to watching films and box sets when I was having treatment for cancer. An awesome and easygoing way to spend a night in. Film Club essentially works the same as a book club.

Get a group together, you all take it in turns to pick a film and discus what you loved or loathed about the film at the end. My only advice would be, make sure that you are watching uplifting, happy or funny movies. Films that are going to lift your spirits otherwise it all just gets too depressing.

TOP TIP

When I found out I had cancer, I asked all my friends to bring their favorite feel-good movie with them so I had lots of lovely things to watch over the coming months (another good thing when people ask what they can do to help), which I would also recommend doing.

There are companies such as Amazon Prime and Netflix, where you pay a monthly subscription and you can stream films through the internet. You need a Smart TV or a device such as a PlayStation that is connected to your internet and the TV for them to work.

BOOK CLUB

Just like with the Film Club... Get your friends who enjoy books together. Meet around once a month, each month a different person picks a book, you all read that book and the following month get together again to talk about it. Someone else picks a book, and so on. It needn't cost any money either, join your local library and take them out for free. Again, I would stick with the uplifting stories.

You could get people to come to you, ask them to bring drinks and nibbles, or share the load and take it in turns for members to host.

If you like the idea but aren't sure about starting an actual book club, there are now a lot online. There is the Richard and Judy Book Club, and most of the women's monthly magazines have one.

PARTY PLANNING PARTY

Remember the old-fashioned tupperwear parties? Well they have moved on so much now and you seem to be able to find a company that sells everything. From beauty products to jewellery to clothes to cookware there is a party that you will like.

How it Works

Invite your friends, family and neighbors to come over to your home. A consultant from your chosen company comes to the house, does a 'show' or 'party' and then everyone has the option to buy the products the consultant has demonstrated. As the host of the party it is usual for to get a gift from the consultant and free products depending on the levels of sales from the party. The company consultant will be able to explain more about this.

I have listed a couple of suggestions below based on what type of products you like:

- ❖ Jewellery – Stella and Dot
- ❖ Skincare – Neal's Yard Remedies Organic
- ❖ Kitchen ware – The Pampered Chef
- ❖ Lingerie – Ann Summers
- ❖ Fashion – Captain Tourtue (Could be a fantastic option if you want to revamp your wardrobe)
- ❖ Make-Up and Cosmetics - Avon

USEFUL LINKS

www.amazon.co.uk/Prime

www.netflicks.com

www.richardandjudy.co.uk

www.stellaanddot.co.uk

www.pamperedchef.co.uk

www.annsummers.com

www.avonshop.co.uk

www.en.captaintortuegroup.com

www.nyrorgnic.co.uk

Chapter Seven

CHANGING LOOKS,
IT'S ALL ABOUT THE CONFIDENCE

A Woman should be two things,
classy and fabulous
- Coco Channel

Oh confidence. You little monkey, you! One minute you are there, the next you have vanished – along with the ability to smell fried mushrooms without wanting to vomit. Physical changes are an inevitable part of cancer treatment. There is a high chance that after your operation you are going to feel and look different. Whether it is because you have lost a breast, gained a colostomy bag or have visible scarring, it can all have an effect on your confidence and those changes can mean that your current wardrobe isn't working for you.

I was left with a permanent colostomy bag after the

operation to remove all the cancerous cells from my colon and surrounding areas, which is attached to the left side of my stomach, at the same height as my belly button. Before the operation, I tended to wear fitted tops and skinny jeans. After my operation I found it very hard to dress. Clothes that were loose around the waist and hid the colostomy bag made me feel like I was wearing a tent. It wasn't made any easier by the fact that I wasn't feeling well enough to be traipsing around the shops.

Every time I opened my wardrobe my heart would sink as I looked at all these gorgeous clothes that I had accumulated over the years, including some which held special meanings to me or had been passed down to me from my late mother. I was devastated that I wouldn't get to wear them again. Getting dressed became a nightmare because I would spend the whole time looking at what I wanted to be wearing and feeling sorry for myself.

TOP TIP

Do not stand in front of the mirror examining every aspect of your body imagining what it would be like if it hadn't changed. You will drive yourself crazy, trust me!

Eventually I decided it was time to take control of the situation, starting with a major clear out.

CLEAR OUT YOUR WARDROBE

I have heard, many times before, that you should clear out your wardrobe once and year and throw out anything you haven't worn in the last two years. I have never done this! As a result the prospect of clearing it out was a huge and daunting task, but here are some ways to make it fun!

Fashion Show

Get your partner, a friend, sister or anyone whose opinion you trust, round to your house and put on a fashion show. Think *Sex in the City* when Carrie gets all the girls round for champagne and to help her pack her wardrobe.

It will make it more fun having the support there, but more importantly, changes to your body can feel like it did when you were a teenager with a spot on the end of your nose. You feel like there is a bright red beacon shouting 'look how awful I look,' but in reality, no one else even notices. So a second opinion is always a good idea.

Try everything on and split it into one of three piles – keep, sell and chuck. Now, if I was being particularly fantastic, I would take the opportunity to put everything I am keeping back neatly and organised. Opening your wardrobe is now a joy and you can see all your gorgeous clothes, which you know you look fabulous in!

OUT WITH THE OLD & IN WITH THE NEW

There is a saying that one woman's trash is another woman's treasure, and this is definitely true of clothes. Since having a colostomy I find myself looking at clothes I wouldn't have considered before. I remember my sister came round wearing a beautiful loose fitted jumper that I thought would suit me perfectly now. I asked her where she bought it and of course she couldn't remember (and it didn't have a tag inside - random), but a few weeks later my sister brought it over, saying that she hardly wore it so I could have it (yay). I know that I have clothes that my sister or friends would look great in that I will never wear now, so it seems like a good time for a clothes swap!

Swishing Party

Basically, you pick a date, invite your friends, colleagues, neighbours or whoever you think would be best suited, around to your house. Everyone brings clothes they no longer want, you check out everyone else's clothes and get to choose which ones you like.

TOP TIP

Think about how big your place is when you are inviting people to the party. There is no point inviting fifty people if you can only fit ten in your house.

Let guests know that clothes must be in good condition and that you get to take the same amount of clothes as you bring, so the more you bring, the more new clothes you get to take home!

On the Night

❖ Have a set time for guests to arrive and drop off clothes.

❖ Clothes can be quickly checked and your guest is given a voucher letting them know what they can pick (how you do this is up to you and I have given some suggestions below).

❖ All items are then put on display so that guests can have a look and ideally try them on before the official 'swish' is open.

❖ Open the Swish!

There are a variety of ways you can swish and it really comes down to which you prefer…

Go For It

Guests can pick the same number of items they have bought. If they've brought ten items they can pick any other ten items. Done.

Fairs Fair

Have three piles: 'bargain', 'mid range' and 'expensive'. When guests arrive they put their items in the correct pile and get a corresponding colour ticket, which they write their name on the back of.

When the swish opens, everyone puts their tickets in a bowel and someone picks the tickets out one-by-one. If the first ticket says 'Nicola' and it's an expensive colour, Nicola can choose an item from the expensive rack. And so the cycle continues.

Best of Both

This is my favourite. Have two drop off points and everyone is given a corresponding ticket. When the swish is open, everyone picks his or her first item. When everyone has chosen, guests get to pick their second item and so on until each person has run out of tickets.

Any items that are left over can be donated to the charity shop.

TOP TIP

If you would like a swishing party but you don't feel up to running it yourself, you could always ask that person who keeps offering to help if they could host it for you.

If you don't want to host your own swishing party, there are organised parties all over the UK on a regular basis that you can go along to. Check out www.swish.com or www.bigwardrobe.com for details of their next events.

SELL, SELL, SELL

There is one obvious thing you need in the quest to revamp your wardrobe, money! What better way to come by it than by selling clothes you are no longer going to wear.

It's not just about EBay anymore; although that is of course an option, there are now a number of websites dedicated to selling second hand clothes.

Here are some ideas:

Vinted

Perfect for High Street labels, with Vinted you can sell, swap, buy or give away your stylish second-hand clothes, shoes, and accessories. The site is easily laid out and so far has avoided being used as a marketplace by sellers. www.vinted.co.uk

Preloved

Preloved is great because it is free to list. Again a good range of labels and styles of clothes, from wedding dresses to high street t-shirts. You can also sell other household items. It's useable and easy to navigate. www.preloved.co.uk

Buy My Wardrobe

If you have high-end designer clothes then it may be worth using a high-end resale site and Buy My Wardrobe is fantastic. The commission is higher but clothes should also sell for more.

The other great thing about Buy My Wardrobe is

that they offer a consignment service, saving you any of the hassle. You send then a list of the items you have for sale by e-mail and when requested, you drop off your items or arrange for a collection. They will take and upload the photos and answer any queries and you will get paid when the items are sold.

www.buymywardrobe.com

SHOPPING

It can be strange shopping after a bodily change. I remember wishing I could have Gok Wan to '*Gok*' me (I actually even went online trying to find out how you get on 'How to Look Good Naked.') But in the absence of someone who would have inevitably been upset when I refused to get naked (colostomy bag or no colostomy bag, it's not happening) you will have to find a style and outfits that you are happy with and that work for your body now, even if it takes a little while.

TOP TIP

My husband said that buying me a few new clothes was a way that he felt he could do something to cheer me up. It made him feel useful knowing that he could do something to help that would make me feel better.

If you are feeling nervous about being in a changing room, you can take someone with you to stand outside the room, making sure staff aren't coming in and out. They can also help with collecting different sizes and giving opinions.

GIVE YOURSELF A BREAK

*Once again and most importantly – **be kind to yourself.** You have been through an incredible change, and you are probably still in the midst of major upheaval. Give yourself time and allow things to settle.*

HAIR TODAY, GONE TOMORROW

Not all types of chemotherapy will make you lose your hair. Mine didn't, so I can only imagine if you *are* losing your hair how you must be feeling.

As I didn't go through it, I didn't feel like I am best placed to talk about it and do it justice, so let me introduce my friend Emma who did lose her hair when having treatment for Breast Cancer when she was 27;

Losing my hair to chemotherapy was almost worse than the cancer itself. I could hide the caner, but hair is the first thing that people see. When I went out, it screamed,

"Look at me, I'm ill." I was 27 when I was diagnosed with grade three-breast cancer. I had noticed a lump when I was nursing my daughter but put it down to the usual changes in the breasts whilst breast-feeding. Six months later, the lump hadn't disappeared so I decided to see my GP. I was referred for tests but I never expected it to be cancer. When I found it was in fact cancer, it took a while for the news to actually sink in.

As tough as I knew the chemotherapy would be, there was one way I thought I could take control – cut my hair off before it fell out. I booked an appointment with my hairdresser and my long straight brown hair was replaced with a short, funky cut that I loved.

It was around this time that I met Jasmin Gupta, a hairdresser who runs the charity *Cancer Hair Care*. In our sessions together she removed a lot of my fear, as well as helping me with the practical side of losing my hair, like getting my wig fashionably cut, to teaching me how to tie head scarves, to suggesting oils for encouraging hair re-growth.

Still, when my hair did start coming out in patches a few weeks after my first chemotherapy treatment (at a big work conference) I was in shock. The smallest tug caused a handful of hair to come out. I didn't want to go outside, as I truly thought the wind would blow away my hair. Finding the right hats, scarves and a wig that I thought *looked natural was great, as that meant I didn't have to explain the cancer to everyone I met, but I still felt ugly and as if all my femininity and beauty had been stolen from me.*

It wasn't until about a month after I finished my chemotherapy during a holiday to Tenerife with my family that I found the confidence to take off my hat in public. I remember getting into the pool, terrified, feeling that I had a huge flashing siren over my head. While it was one of the scariest things I've ever done, it was also one of the most liberating and it felt like a real breakthrough moment.

Gradually, over the next few months my hair started to grow back. It was darker and coarser than before but it was growing. As soon as my hair was long enough to colour, I decided I wanted to make a statement, to show I was back in control of my looks. I bought a home colouring kit and dyed my hair bright red. Over five years later, I am in remission, my hair is no longer bright red but I've keep my hair short, it's who I am now.

Emma, Breast Cancer, 27

Cancer Hair Care

One of the best resources that I have come across with regards to hair loss is the amazing Cancer Hair Care charity that Emma spoke about in her piece above. Their website is full of video tutorials, resources, links and a helpline. If you are losing or have lost you hair, it is certainly worth taking a look. www.cancerhaircare.com

USEFUL CONTACTS

www.cancerhaircare.com
www.vinted.co.uk
www.preloved.co.uk
www.buymywardrobe.com
www.swish.com
www.bigwardrobe.com

Chapter Eight

WELL DESERVED REST & RELAXATION

Let her sleep, for when she wakes,
She will move mountains.
- Napoleon

I love this quote because it truly encapsulates what you are doing, allowing yourself to build strength during the biggest fight of your life.

It's not always easy but taking time for yourself is more important than ever when you are going through cancer. You need to allow your body and mind to recharge and restore whenever you can.

SLEEP

I found when I had a chemotherapy session, it would take so much out of me physically that my sleep would actually improve for that week. However, the rest of the time my sleep was often interrupted with worry or physical discomfort.

For me, the worst part of sleep deprivation is how emotional it would leave me feeling over the next day or so. I always find it harder to cope when I am tired, I become snappy, tearful and it is all just *horrible*. So trying to stay on top of sleep is very important.

These are the things I tried to do to help me sleep:

❖ **Avoid caffeine or anything stimulating in the afternoon.**
   This includes soft drinks, especially fizzy soft drinks, which tend to be high in sugar and contain caffeine.

❖ **Try to avoid alcohol.**
   Alcohol seems like a good idea at the time doesn't it? It may help you to initially fall asleep but it's often not a restful sleep and you will inevitably wake up through the night. Try and keep alcohol to a minimum or abstain completely when you are having difficulty sleeping.

❖ **Keep your bedroom clean, uncluttered and dark.**
   This isn't always easy when you are in your room

a lot, particularly post-surgery but do your best, or make it a job for someone who is offering to help. There are more details on keeping your room as your 'Boudoir Sanctuary' at the end of chapter 4, 'Doctors and Hospitals' but if you need a quick reminder:

○ Keep your room clean and tidy.
○ Open a window at least once a day, even if it is only for a few minutes, to keep the fresh air circulating.
○ Get someone to change your sheets every few days. Decadent yes, but trust me, you will feel so much better for it.
○ Flowers always brighten a room!
○ Display photo's that will keep you uplifted, inspired and remind you what you are fighting for.

❖ **Use lavender essential oil.**

Just pop a couple of drops on your pillow or onto a handkerchief so that you can gently inhale the oil to help you fall asleep. Lavender is a great oil to have in your cancer toolkit because it is useful for so many things.

❖ **Sleep meditation CD's.**

I would spend whole weeks using sleep meditation CD's every night and I swear by them when you can't sleep. They work so well because rather than lying there in silence thinking about how you can't sleep, you focus on the CD.

My favourite sleep meditation was one I downloaded from iTunes called 'Best Sleep Meditation' by Moments of Magic.

❖ **Send light through your body to relax your muscles.**

I do this all the time if I can't sleep. Imagine that there is a white light coming in through the top of your scalp, relaxing every muscle it touches. Start right at the top of your scalp, mentally relaxing every muscle with the white light and work your way down all through your body to your toes.

Personally I am often (not always) asleep well before I get to my toes. Just really take your time with it, feeling and relaxing every single muscle. Remember to do the front and the back of your body.

❖ **Don't get frustrated if you only sleep in short spurts.**

This is very normal. When your body is under this much strain, it needs to recharge every few hours rather than going the sixteen hours (or so) you would go between sleeps in a normal sleep pattern. It may result in you sleeping for short spurts during the day too, but this is normal and what your body needs.

❖ **Give yourself a break.**
   If I could underline this fifteen times, I would. Your sleep is going to be affected by something like cancer. Getting stressed by it will inevitably make it worse, so give yourself a break and don't let going to sleep become a moment in your day that you dread.

TOP SLEEP TIP

FROM MY ONCOLOGY NURSE

If you can't sleep, or only sleep in short spurts, that's fine. Keep sleep in perspective. Just relax and let your body rest. There will be plenty of time to re-set your sleep pattern once this difficult time is over, but for now, just sleep when and as often as you can.

MEDITATION

Honestly, meditation is not just for the hippies and Buddhists of the world, it really is fantastic for everyone. It can take a while to get used to meditating and get the technique down to a fine art.

I mentioned meditation CDs when talking about sleep in the 'sleep' section (page 111), but you can meditate at any time of the day. I know women who meditate first thing in the morning to set themselves up for the day and in the afternoon to give them a recharge for the afternoon and evening, so whatever suits you will be perfect.

As I said, you can meditate using a CD, which is particularly useful if you struggle to stop your thoughts intruding. It means you can focus on the worlds and the music of the CD. This combined with the specific nature of the hypnotic words should soothe you into a relaxed state.

You can also meditate on your own, which can allow you to settle into a deeper meditative state as you 'switch off' altogether.

How to Meditate On Your Own
❖ **Set aside some time.**
If you haven't meditated before, you only want to start with setting aside five to fifteen minutes to mediate in.

❖ **Create a quiet, calming environment.**
You don't want anything to distract you or break your attention whilst meditating so turn off the TV, put your mobile on silent and unplug the landline.

You can play music but make sure it is on quietly and that it is calm and repetitive so it does not distract you. You don't want to realise you are singing along to Kylie and not switching off at all.

❖ **Sit or lie comfortably.**
Do not worry about getting into any strange positions – this isn't an endurance or flexibility task. Sitting or lying

comfortably is perfect.

If you are sitting, sit on the edge of a cushion, this will tilt your pelvis forward a touch and be more comfortable. The main thing is to remember is to keep your back straight. Starting from the base of your spine, imagine stacking each vertebra directly on top of the one below. Start at the bottom of your back and go all the way up to your head. This ensures your lungs have more space and you can breath easily and deeply.

If you are lying down, bend your knees slightly, or pop a pillow underneath you knees. This will also tip your pelvis slightly and straighten your spine. I personally find it *so* much more comfortable with my knees bent a touch.

Ultimately, just make sure you are comfortable.

❖ **Relax your body.**

Close your eyes and focus on your body. Mentally scan your body, looking for any points that are tense and consciously relax them with your mind. Remember to check your face, neck and scalp too.

You might then need to adjust your position slightly and straighten out again when you have finished.

❖ **Rest your attention on the flow of your breath.**

Listen to your breath, but try not to think about it. For example thinking, "My breath is very quick, I need it to calm down, why won't it calm down," is clearly not going to make you calm. Don't judge it; just let it fall into a natural rhythm. Let all the 'noise' from your mind fade away as you concentrate on this one thing.

As a beginner you can count your breath from one to ten and then start at number one again to give you *something* to focus on.

❖ Silence your mind.

The final step is clearing you mind by focusing on nothing at all. This is the pinnacle of meditation and it can take a while to reach this point (I have never got there) but it is what you are eventually aiming for.

If a thought does pop into your head, don't panic or think you have failed at meditating. Just picture the thought floating away from your mind, without thinking about it or judging it, like a balloon. Then re-centre yourself and carry on.

Take the same approach with any thoughts that come into your mind until only silence prevails.

❖ Remember

It takes practice to focus and clear you mind. Don't expect your mind to be completely silent the first time. Meditation is a non-judgemental process. If you can do mediate straight away, great, if you can't, that's fine too. You will still feel a benefit from five minutes of quiet breathing and re-centring yourself. Allow yourself time to learn this skill and just enjoy the journey.

> *TOP TIPS FOR MEDITATING*
>
> *If you find it difficult to meditate for the time you have allowed yourself, try a shorter time. Try just one or two minutes to begin with.*
>
> *It is not advised to meditate for longer than thirty minutes in one go. If you want to meditate for longer, try introducing a second session into your day.*
>
> *See if you notice a difference in your general mood or sleep patterns on the day's you meditate and note any improvements.*

WRITE IT DOWN

Journaling or keeping a diary is often considered a fantastic way to relax and unwind as it can allow you to expel any negative thoughts and worries. Writing down stressful times and events can be a good way to come to terms with what is happening, clarifying your thoughts and feelings and release the intensity of them.

Keeping a diary also helps you to notice patterns in your emotions. As I said in chapter five, 'The Emotional Roller-Coaster,' something I learnt was the concept that 'this too shall pass'. As I identified patterns in my emotions, I was able to prepare myself for when they came round again and not to let them overwhelm me.

How to Start Writing

A good way to start is to not to worry about punctuation or spelling, don't censor yourself, don't think about what you want to write, just write. There is no right or wrong way to do it. For this purpose, you don't need to worry about what you writing making sense, the sole purpose is just to get the thoughts out, no matter how random or incoherent they are.

When sitting down to write, it can be good to start with a few minutes of 'free writing' as mentioned above, with no planning or forward-thinking, just to get any random thoughts out and then continue with what you would like to write about.

Write to Someone

Some people find it easier if they feel they are writing *to* someone. You could set up another email account and write emails to yourself. Or letters that you never post. You can also keep blog's private if you wish to collate all your messages in one place.

Writing a Narrative

For some, writing through the form of a story or narrative can work very well as it gives a level of detachment to the emotions you are writing about and it can allow you to be a little more reflective.

For example you may write a story about a small girl who has just been diagnosed with cancer and how she tells her friends at school. In doing this you will be able to explore your own feelings of your situation without confronting them head on. You may find yourself giving her advice that you could take yourself.

The wonderful thing about writing is that it can allow you to open and evolve the creative side of your brain, rather than forever staying in the worrying part!

REMEMBER

As you don't have to confide in anyone, you really can release your inner most thoughts. Think of this wonderful quote from Oscar Wilde; "I never travel without my diary. One should always have something sensational to read on the train." I think that says it all.

GO OUTSIDE

I know I have mentioned this in chapter five, The Emotional Rollercoaster but it can be a fantastic way to relax – weather and wellness permitting. You can just sit in the park or the garden.

If you aren't up to going outside or nerve damage is giving you trouble, just push a chair close to an open window to watch the clouds and any birds flying by. It will still have a wonderfully calming effect.

TAKE UP A HOBBY

Apparently, if you can absorb your brain in a simple and repetitive task, it can help you to relax and feel calmer. So, skydiving? Rollerblading? No! Well thankfully I'm not talking about those kinds of hobbies but there are plenty that you can do from the comfort of your own home or bed.

Personally, I am thrilled that adult colouring in is now socially acceptable because I always find it so relaxing colouring in with my daughter and now you can get the most wonderfully intricate designs that you can really become absorbed in. I love it (my life is *so* rock n' roll).

Obviously there is a lot in this book that you could turn into hobbies like meditation or journaling, but here are a few additional ideas:

- ❖ Colouring books – as I said.
- ❖ Knitting
- ❖ Sewing
- ❖ Play games online or on your phone
- ❖ Card games
- ❖ Learn a language with CD's or online.
- ❖ Letters Writing – there is a scheme One Million Lovely Letters that sends letters to people who need cheering up. Or find a pen pal from anywhere in the world through a site such as International Pen Friends. Then you can enjoy getting something through the post other than medical letters and appointment times.

PAMPER PARTY FOR ONE

You have all the details of having a wonderful Pamper Party with your friends in chapter six, 'Staying In and Staying Social' but you don't need everyone round at your house. Take some time to treat yourself and turn your home into an At-Home-Spa.

Enjoy one, two, or all of the pamper party treats on your own, or here are a few additional ideas:

Cleopatra Spa Bath

I am a big fan of a bath, but let's be clear, I don't mean just washing. I mean the ritual of bathing and turning your bathroom into your own little private spa bath.

If you are having the type of chemotherapy that is creating uncomfortable cold in your body and causing nerve damage, Cleopatra's Spa Bath can be particularly soothing but your nerves will be oversensitive when you get out so make sure that you have a big warm towel and dressing gown ready to wrap yourself up in as soon as you get out.

- ❖ Run a bath with your favourite bubble bath, light some candles or tea-lights and pop on some relaxing music.
- ❖ Have an oil burner with four drops of Lavender, two drops of Ylang Ylang and two drops of Frankincense, to make a gorgeous smelling aromatic blend that is very relaxing and calming. Perfect for relaxing in the bath. If you don't

have all these essential oils, just Lavender will be fine.

❖ Sink into the bath letting all your tension dissolve in the warm water, bliss!

TOP TIP

If you don't have an oil burner, you can fill a small bowl or dish with some water and the essential oils and pop it on the radiator, it will have a very similar effect.

Oil burners tend to be very reasonably priced if you would like one.

WARM & NOURISHING SCALP TREATMENT

This is a fantastic hot oil treatment that will treat your hair (which ever stage in your cycle it may be in) and scalp, as we all hold so much tension in our scalp. You could do this before getting in to your Cleopatra Bath for a truly relaxing time.

❖ Warm three tablespoons of olive oil by gently heating it on the hob.

❖ Pour it into a bowl.

❖ If your oncologist agrees to you using essential oils directly onto the skin, add two drops of Rosemary and two drops of Lavender essential oil to the warm olive oil.

❖ Massage the oil into the scalp, coating the oil to the ends of your hair.

❖ Cover your head with a shower cap, then a towel and let the mixture do it's thing for at least fifteen minutes.

❖ Wash it all out.

TOP TIP

You will need to shampoo your hair twice to make sure you wash all of the oil out.

HAVE A HOLISTIC OR BEAUTY TREATMENT

Don't want to do it yourself? Have someone else treat you to a treatment.

ALWAYS

Check with your oncologist before going for any holistic or beauty treatments, even just a massage.

My oncologist said that I couldn't have massage but she was happy for me to have reflexology or a facial, so make sure you check first.

Most beauty or holistic therapists will require a doctors letter stating that they agree to you having treatments so if you are interested, make sure that you get one from someone in your team.

If you are allowed and would like a treatment but don't want to go to a salon or spa, there are now a number of beauty and holistic therapists offering mobile services who can come to your home. They will usually set up their own treatment couch and come with everything they need and take it all away again, so you can just sit back and relax without having to do anything.

Ask around to see if any of your friends can recommend anyone, if not you could try mobile services My Pamper Party or Blossom and Jasmine, who both run with national schemes using local beauty and holistic therapists.

MOST IMPORTANTLY

If any of the suggestions above become another 'thing that you think you need to squeeze in to your already exhausted time' and therefore become stressful…

DO NOT DO THEM.

All of these suggestions (as with the whole book) are meant to make life easier and be coping strategies. The moment they stop making life easier, stop.

You can always come back to it later if you so choose.

USEFUL CONTACTS

www.blossomandjasmine.com
www.mypamperparty.net
www.onemillionlovelyletters.com
www.ipfworld.com

Chapter Nine

DIET & EXERCISE

The only carrots that interest me,
Are the number you get in a diamond
- Mae West

I know, I know, you can't really be bothered, especially right now, but it will be worth it.

Just to be clear, I am not talking about running a marathon or starting your own organic vegetable patch, but some gentle exercise and some extra vitamins and minerals can make all the difference to your general well being and can be especially beneficial when you have cancer.

As well as fighting cancer, diet and exercise are also linked to better sleep, more energy, a stronger immune system, all of which will be beneficial right now.

DIET

You may be thinking, '*I've already got cancer, what good is an anti-cancer diet to me now?*' Well, I am a big believer in throwing everything you can at cancer, in an attempt to beat it into submission, using every possible tool. That can included your diet.

I think that the stronger you can make your body at a time when cancer, chemotherapy, radiotherapy and a whole host of other medication are trying to deplete it, the better. Cancer is a totally selfish sod and will be busy feeding off all that is good in your body and leaving you with the leftover crap, so you need to work extra hard to ensure there is more than just crap remaining. That way, your body will have more strength to fight the cancer and process all the medication.

Diet can also help with keeping your energy levels high and ward off the minor illnesses that you really want to avoid when having treatment. A good diet can also contribute to you healing quicker after an operation. Plus, if you get your diet right now, you should, in theory, have a wonderful anti-cancer diet up and running, ready for after your treatment.

As much as we would all love to be told that the only thing we need to eat is chocolate – it aint going to happen! There is no big secret when it comes to eating well. You know this. You know what you should be eating and avoiding. It's the same thing we always hear; eat less processed food, salt, sugar, ready-meals and fast food and eat more fresh fruit, vegetables, whole grains and pulses.

Why Do I Have to Eat That?

Fruit and vegetables are packed with antioxidants, which 'kill' free radicals. Free radicals are the nasties that can trigger cancer by damaging the DNA in our cells and causing cells to mutate so we want to do everything we can to get rid of them.

Plus – free radicals also cause wrinkles! So as you can see, there really is *every* reason to fight them off.

Fruit and vegetables protect you against all types of cancer so you want to eat as many as possible, ideally a brightly coloured mixture to gain the maximum benefit.

Fibre is also a superhero in the internal fight against cancer.

Insoluble fibre that you find in whole grains, fruit and vegetables pulls the contents of your digestive system through your bowels, reducing the amount of time that cancer causing chemicals called carcinogens spend in contact with your bowel walls.

Soluble fibre that you find in oats, pulses, fruit and vegetables produces friendly bacteria, which then produce chemicals that can help to prevent tumours from developing.

Strengthen Your Immunity

From cancer to the common cold, your body needs strong defences, which means you need to develop a strong immune system.

The immune system is made up of several systems,

plus an 'army' of cells which roam the body looking for trouble to deal with.

IT IS WORTH REMEMBERING

This army can only work effectively in clear conditions, so if your body is polluted with smoke, sugar, processed foods and any other toxins, this army is not going to be able to do its job of finding the nasties and dealing with them properly.

The best immune nutrients are vitamins A, C and E, all the B vitamins, zinc and selenium.

The best sources of these nutrients are:

Vitamin A - meat, eggs, dairy products and oily fish.

Vitamin C - green vegetables, kiwi fruit, blackcurrants, citrus fruits and strawberries.

Vitamin E – nuts (especially almonds), seeds and seed oils such as sunflower oil, eggs and avocados.

B Vitamins – meat, dairy products, eggs, whole grains, pulses, nuts, seeds, green leafy vegetables.

Zinc – lean meat (by far the richest source), seafood, dairy products, chickpeas, pumpkin seeds, sunflower seeds and nuts.

Selenium – Brazil nuts, fish (especially shellfish), kidney and liver.

Fighting Fatigue and Stress

I am seriously guilty of craving and eating huge amounts of sugary snacks, caffeine and some sort of convenient, fast, comfort food when I am feeling stressed or tired. A number of people will also add alcohol to the list. We want a quick fix to how we are feeling don't we? In reality, they are having the opposite effect. They give us a quick pick me up and then before you can say *I probably shouldn't have eaten/drunk that,'* you are back on the floor as the sugar dip descends and you end up feeling even worse. This is not what you need right now, so try and avoid everything mentioned above if possible.

So what should you do to fight fatigue and stress with your diet? Keep nutrient levels high. When you are stressed and tired certain nutrients are quickly drained by your body such as the B vitamins, magnesium and the all-important vitamin C, so you really want to be keeping these nutrients coming into your body.

B Vitamins – meat, dairy products, eggs, whole grains, pulses, nuts, seeds, green leafy vegetables.

Magnesium – almonds, fish and green leafy vegetables such as spinach and kale.

Vitamin C - green vegetables, kiwi fruit, blackcurrants, citrus fruits and strawberries.

GET THESE FOODS IN YOUR DIET

I am not someone who naturally gravitates towards vegetables so they are something I have to actively try and include. I tend to do this by eating normally and hiding as many vegetables in as many dishes as possible (if you are a mum you are probably used to this) but for me this includes things like adding kale to spaghetti bolognese and a layer of spinach between the potatoes and meat in a shepherds pie, that sort of thing.

Having said that, you may find that your appetite isn't what it was before you had cancer, which is why I cannot suggest soups and juices enough because they are such an excellent way of getting fabulous nutrients into your body, when you don't feel like you want to eat.

Here are a few quick and easy ways I found to get as much healthy stuff as possible into my body through juices and soups:

TOP TIP

Chemotherapy often changes your taste buds. You may find foods you didn't like before now taste lovely and visa versa, so it is worth giving new things a try, you never know; you may now love Brussels sprouts!

JUICING & BLENDING

First things first, the difference between juicing and blending:

Juicing - you put your fruit or vegetables into the juicer and it squeezes every last piece of juice out, leaving only the pulp behind. Juicing is fantastic for hard vegetables like carrots and hard fruits like apples.

Blending - the blades chop the entire fruit and vegetable until it becomes a juice. Blending is perfect for soft fruit and vegetables like spinach, kale, berries and bananas.

I have both but personally I prefer using the blender. It is a lot quicker and easier to clean. The benefit of using a blender is that because everything is blended, including the skin, all the fibre is kept, whereas fibre is usually lost when using a juicer. Having said that, I know other people who swear by their juicers so it's all about whatever works best for you and which one you prefer.

Juicing and blending are fantastic for you at the moment because when you are having chemotherapy it can be hard to keep your appetite and this way you are still getting all those important nutrients that are found in vegetables.

Mixing fruit and vegetables means that you will get the natural sweetness from the fruit and can make a gorgeous drink, packed with everything you need to give your body a boost. Antioxidants found in fruit and vegetables are reported to work effectively when they are consumed together so mix away.

Some scientists say that the actual act of eating fruit and vegetables mean that your body absorbs more of the nutritional content in healthy foods so I wouldn't live on juices alone (I physically couldn't even if I wanted to) but remember that you are living in extreme circumstances and better that you are getting some nutrition rather than nothing at all.

Here are a couple of seriously easy juice recipes to get you started...

The Green One

❖ *A large handful of spinach*

❖ *Half a cucumber*

❖ *1 or 2 celery sticks*

❖ *Half a small pineapple*

❖ *Splash of still water – you can substitute this for coconut water if you like.*

Cut the cucumber, celery sticks and pineapple into chunks. Chuck everything in the blender, spinach first. Blend and drink. You can keep any leftover in the fridge for a day or so but it does always taste better when first blended.

> ## TOP TIP
>
> *Keep spinach in the freezer. Spinach tends to wilt quickly in the fridge, this way it will keep for much longer. The leaves stay separate and crispy and it makes the juice lovely and cold. No need to defrost, pop it straight in.*

The Orange One

- ❖ *1 carrot*
- ❖ *2 small apples*

Core the apples and cut the top off the carrot. Pop in the juicer and bobs-your-uncle, a delicious, sweet and healthy drink. This is an easily drinkable drink so can be a good one to start juicing with.

The Red One

- ❖ *200g raw beetroot*
- ❖ *1 large orange*
- ❖ *Handful of spinach*

Blend the beetroot and spinach, squeeze out and add the orange juice.

The Purple One

- ❖ *Handful of strawberries*
- ❖ *Handful of blackberries*
- ❖ *Handful of blueberries*
- ❖ *1 small banana*
- ❖ *A small handful of spinach or kale*
- ❖ *Optional extra – a large splash of Almond Milk, will make it a little creamer*

Peel the banana but other than that, you just chuck everything in a blender and blend. A yummy, delicious, sweet juice.

TOP TIP

You can use frozen berries, again they will keep for much longer and most supermarkets do frozen bags of mixed berries. No need to defrost, you can drop them straight in and blend away.

SOUPS

The great thing about soup is that you can still enjoy them if your chemotherapy is giving you nerve damage so you can't have cold or room temperature drinks.

Here are my two easiest ones:

The Chicken One

- ❖ *A whole, small chicken*
- ❖ *6 peeled carrots*
- ❖ *4 celery stalks*
- ❖ *1 onion*
- ❖ *Any other vegetable's you feel like adding*

In a large saucepan, pop in the whole chicken, half the carrots and celery stalks cut into chunky pieces and a quarter of the onion. Cover all the ingredients with cold water, bring to the boil and then reduce to a simmer for thirty-minutes or until the chicken is cooked through.

Lift the chicken out (carefully) and let it cool. Strain the broth into a bowl, getting rid of the leftover vegetables and pop the broth back into the pan, along with the remaining carrots and celery stalks which are cut into bite size pieces. Simmer for five - ten minutes.

Pull all the chicken off the bone, shredding it into pieces and add to the soup. Done!

The Vegetable One

The great thing about vegetable soup is that you can tailor it to include the vegetables you like, or the ones leftover in your fridge that you need to use up!

- ❖ *200g of raw vegetables of your choice*
- ❖ *300g of potatoes or sweet potatoes if you want to make it healthier*
- ❖ *700ml of vegetable stock*
- ❖ *A splash of oil*

Pop a little oil in a saucepan, add the chopped vegetables and potatoes for two – three minutes and gently sauté, so they start to soften. Cover with stock and simmer for ten – fifteen minutes, until the vegetables are tender.

Chuck it all in the blender and blend until smooth. You can serve with a little crème fraiche to make it creamier if you want to.

Both soups can be kept in the freezer for up to a month, so this could be another great job for someone who is offering to help. They can make a batch and then you can freeze it in individual portions. Yum!

ASK THE EXPERTS

Thankfully there is now a wealth of information when it comes to eating 'clean' and healthily both online and in the bookshops.

My favourite websites for you to check out are:

The Fairy Food Mother, also known as Lauren Gayfer, is a highly qualified nutritional therapist. Lauren's website includes plenty of fabulous and easy recipes that are regularly updated and often with busy women and mums in mind.

www.laurengayfer.co.uk

Ella Woodward is the lady behind the blogging sensation, **Deliciously Ella**. Ella has a great recipe book but there is still mountains of information and delicious recipes on her website – even a healthy version of Nutella, which is my kind of healthy eating!

www.deliciouslyella.com

Honestly Healthy Food was founded by Natasha Corrette who believes in an Alkaline diet for healthy living. Again she has a cookbook but also plenty of information and recipes on her website. I can't lie, this diet plan is not for the faint hearted but you can get some really great healthy ideas, including even more chocolate spread!

www.honestlyhealthyfood.com

EXERCISE

I know, I know, you can't really be bothered with this either, but I promise just a little bit will be worth it. Gentle exercise can really help lift your spirits, keep depression at bay and help to keep your body healthy (relatively of course – this is obviously ignoring the cancer) and strong.

Benefits of Exercise

I am sure that you already know all of this but exercise can help you sleep better, lift your mood, lower your chance of developing heart problems and some cancers, as well as helping your muscles, bones and joints stay strong.

I think the benefits of exercise for cancer specifically are all of the above plus, because you may be spending quite a bit of time sedentary, getting your body moving can be fantastic release to your tired and scrunched up muscles and ligaments. It honestly used to feel like I was breathing life back into my body when I just did some gentle stretches.

Here, the rather fabulous Alice talks about her love for exercise and how it helped her get through not one, but two bouts of cancer:

Exercise was and is a big thing for me. It's my way of getting away from life for a short time, de-stressing and in a bizarre way, relaxing.

When I was diagnosed with cancer a 2nd time I knew running would be the last thing my treatment would allow. For some it is possible to continue but not for me. I dealt with this by aiming to get out for a walk as often as possible. Visiting new places and having new things to look at, as I enjoyed my walk, was very therapeutic for me. Often I would walk with others if I wasn't well enough to be on my own. It really kept me going and lifted my mood immensely.

Some days I couldn't manage it and they were a struggle. I would get depressed but I'd try to focus on the future and plan ways in which I would regain my fitness, looking at events like park run and a local mile run as something to aim for. I also worked with a personal trainer who'd been through cancer herself and she built me back up very gradually.

Exercise for me was and still is very important to keep me mentally healthy as well as physically and in 2015, I fulfilled my dream of successfully running the London Marathon, raising money for Cancer Research UK, of course.

Alice, Hodgkin's Lymphoma, 27
and Ewing's Sarcoma, 37

Before You Start

You need to listen you your body, don't overexert yourself or push things too hard. Always get advice from your GP or oncologist on what would be an appropriate form of exercise. Make sure your mind-set is realistic. If you know you only have a little energy don't try for a hard two-hour session in the gym.

Here are a few exercise suggestions:

Walking – Alice has already talked about this and I agree, it is the most fantastic exercise when you are ill. Walking helps with the blues and depression, I also find emotionally that walking is so fantastic because I am often able to sort my thoughts when I am walking, which for some reason is much harder when cooped up indoors. My chemotherapy meant I couldn't expose my skin to cold so it would take ages during the winter to get wrapped up in scarfs, hats and balaclavas (I kid you not, I actually used to walk through the park with a balaclava on), but even on the days when I could only walk to the end of the road and back, it was worth it. Just that little stretch of my legs would make me feel so much better. So if nothing else, get some comfy shoes on and walk to the end of the road and back.

Running – Same rules as walking apply but running is harder on your joints and muscles so I would build up to it and remember to take it easy. If it feels too much, just walk and try running again at a later date.

Dance – The best thing about dance is that it does not feel like exercise. You don't have to find an adult dance class, just stick some of your favourite tunes on a playlist and go wild around the living room with the kids (which they will love) I can guarantee you will feel better for it.

Swimming – I am always being told it is one of the best forms of exercise, working every muscle group but I never really got it. That was until I had cancer! Every muscle is gently stretched and you have the support of the water. Feels amazing.

Gardening – Yes it does actually count, as long as you are getting stuck in. Unfortunately pruning a couple of roses off a bush doesn't count. I remember cutting back a large hedge with some massive sheers, I was *exhausted* by the time I finished and that was before I knew I had cancer.

Yoga – When I had cancer, I found Yoga amazing. I went to a series of therapeutic yoga classes at the Wallace Cancer Centre in Cambridge when I was in treatment. I have been to yoga classes before and these cancer yoga classes are more easy-going than normal one's, as the focus is to just let you muscles and joints release and stretch, which feels *so* good.

I would recommend speaking with you local cancer centre (pages 17 – 19) and see if they offer yoga because if they do, it will be tailored specifically for people with cancer.

If not, contact your local yoga teacher, explain your situation and see what they say about you attending their class. If their class wouldn't be appropriate, they may be able to recommend someone else who can.

USEFUL CONTACTS

www.laurengayfer.co.uk
www.deliciouslyella.com
www.honestlyhealthyfood.com
www.parkrun.org.uk
www.spotify.com
www.swimming.org/poolfinder
www.yogaclicks.com

Chapter Ten

HOLIDAYS & TRAVEL

Paris, is always a good idea.
- Audrey Hepburn

If you fancy getting away during a suitable break in your treatment, it should be possible. Speak with your oncologist to make sure they are happy for you to go away and that you are at a good point in your treatment programme to do so and I certainly wouldn't book anything until you have absolutely got the OK from your oncologist, but lets face it, I bet no one needs a holiday as much as you and yours do right now!

BEFORE YOU BOOK

The way my treatment worked out meant that I was going to have a six-week break between finishing radiotherapy and my operation. My husband and I were keen to get away and forget the whole cancer debacle for a week or so but I was *very* nervous at the thought of being so far away from my oncological team and hospital that I had come to know so well. What if something happened? What if I contracted a life-threatening infection? What if I burst into flames? All completely rational possibilities.

I spoke to my oncologist and he reassured me that it would be fine and that this was a very suitable pause in my treatment to go on holiday. He advised visiting nearby Europe, ideally a country with a good healthcare system and to make sure that I got an EHIC (which used to be known as the E11) so that I could be treated in a European hospital with no problems should I get ill or something go wrong.

As I have said before, your oncologist is the person to ask if you want to get away, only they can really make sure you are doing everything right.

TOP TIP

Plan ahead. There may be a little more to think about when going on holiday now, so give yourself time to do just that. It will make for a more relaxing holiday in the long run.

WHERE TO GO

I was recommended Western Europe because they accept the EHIC card (more details below) and have good health care systems should anything happen and you need medical attention.

Depending on the type of cancer you have, it may be worth thinking about cultural norms such as the types of food and drink that will be easily accessible. If you have any special dietary requirements can they be easily catered for? Can you drink the water? Does it matter if you can't?

Think about the type of holiday you would like to go on. What once seemed fabulous might not be the right holiday for you at the moment. I love sightseeing, but the type of holiday I needed during my treatment was going to have to be a strictly chilled-out one. I was not going to have the energy for anything else. So take a moment to think and be honest with yourself about what you could realistically cope with at the moment.

I would also take into account the length of the flight should you need to get home quickly and how often airlines fly between your chosen destination and the UK. The last thing you need is to get home quickly whilst feeling ill and not be able to. If you are sticking to Western Europe this shouldn't be too much of a problem but it is still probably best to check.

> ### REMEMBER
>
> *Needing emergency medical attention or to fly home urgently are worst-case scenarios. I don't want to make you nervous, but I equally don't want you to get caught out in a difficult position where you don't speak the language, can't remember the names of key doctor's, can't get treatment because you don't have insurance or an EHIC card and it is going to take you fifty-eight hours to get home.*
>
> *I know that the more prepared you can be, the more confident you will be going away, which is why you should factor all these things into your decision. Then you can go on holiday relaxed, knowing that if something does go wrong, you are covered.*
>
> *As always - Expect the best. Prepare for the worst.*

If you are on a lot of medication or need a constant oxygen tank, anything like that, I would double-check with the airline and the country that you want to visit that there are no restrictions on taking those supplies with you.

WHAT IS AN EHIC?

It stands for European Health Insurance Card, and it enables the owner to receive state-provided healthcare anywhere within the European Economic Area (EEA) for free or at a reduced cost. This includes pre-existing conditions so if there was a problem to do with having cancer it should still be covered.

However, it is not an alternative to travel insurance and as it only covers state-provided healthcare. It wouldn't include transporting you back to the UK, stolen property, anything along those lines. You will still need travel insurance for that.

An EHIC card is free of charge and you apply for an EHIC card from the NHS website, where they also have a wealth of information on what is and isn't covered in various countries by the EHIC. Visit www.nhs.uk/NHSEngland/Healthcareabroad/EHIC

TRAVEL INSURANCE

This is not as easy at it used to be. When you have cancer, insurance companies will not be so desperate to take your money because you might actually make a claim! I can tell you from the outset, you are unlikely to get travel insurance to go to the USA or on a cruise because of the cost of treatment or flying you from a ship to a nearby county, insurance companies just won't risk it. It will be a real-life case of 'computer says no!'

You probably won't be able to apply online. Once you click 'yes' to having cancer, they are going to want to speak to you.

JUST TO PREPARE YOU

The insurance company will ask a lot of questions about your illness, including prognosis (whether its terminal or not) and treatment details, when trying to assess how likely you are to make a claim. It can be upsetting running through everything, especially if they then decide they won't insure you.

Be as upfront as possible because if something happens and they think you should have told them and didn't, they could void your insurance policy and pay nothing!

There are specialist insurance companies who provide cancer-related insurance but the premiums will be higher. Alternatively, you may get an insurance quote that covers non-cancer related claims. So if you had to cancel your trip because your cancer has made you too ill to travel, that wouldn't be covered. It's up to you which way to go.

The price comparison site Money Supermarket has a 'travel insurance when you have cancer' filter so you can do an initial search but then you will probably need to speak to your favourite companies directly to get a clear idea of costs and what is covered in the plan.

STAYCATION

Of course you don't have to go abroad. Our little island is bursting with wonderful places to visit and what better time to do it than when you can't be bothered with the hassle of going away.

We have award-winning beaches in Dorset, seal watching off the Norfolk coast, Bath just being the fabulous Bath, the Eden Project and Lizard Peninsula in Cornwall, the Yorkshire Dales, The Fringe Festival in Edinburgh, the beauty of the Lake District, travelling by train on the Snowdon mountain railway... the list goes on and on.

I can't guarantee you good weather but I can guarantee an NHS hospital relatively nearby!

Take a look Visit England's website for inspiration about what you can get up to without travelling abroad. www.visitengland.com

BEFORE YOU GO

Even when the holiday was booked and my oncologist was happy, I was still *so* nervous. Just to clarify I was going to France with my husband, toddler and baby to visit my in-laws who live there and the medical care in France is great. This was not a dramatic holiday, nevertheless I was still so nervous.

Looking back I realise worry is what you would expect to feel at this point, but I could also weigh my nervousness against the need (and want) for a break from everything – holiday won!

If you are also experiencing a momentary panic, don't worry, just weigh up the options in your own circumstance and come to a decision that you and your oncologist are happy with.

TOP TIP

Being as organised as possible will help with nerves. Think about every part of the trip and what you may need. Check for local hospitals so that if anything happens you have all the information to hand and you won't be scrambling around for an internet connection and translating pages to find out where the hospital is.

One of the wonderful things about the internet is with sites like www.tripadvisor.com you are able to fully investigate an area before you go. If there is anywhere in particular you want to visit, eat at or deliberately avoid, you can check it all out. You can be as meticulous as you like, so you feel as confident as possible arriving at your destination.

WHAT TO PACK

Oh my goodness, this is hard enough at the best of times, let alone when you have cancer. I will assume that clothes, swimming cozzie and toothbrush are a given and you know to pack those.

❖ Take a copy of your doctor's notes or you can get a letter from your GP highlighting the key facts and details including an up-to-date list of medications.

❖ Take contact details of your oncology team in the UK including names, extensions, your NHS number and your hospital number so that the medical team on holiday can contact your medical team in the UK easily, should they need too. Or if you have a question whilst you are out there, you can contact them easily.

❖ Keep thinking about how your current state will be when you are away. For example, if you are still feeling the side effects of chemotherapy like mouth ulcers make sure you take your cream. If you are still feeling nerve damage, take warm booties, gloves and so forth because even in hot countries, evenings can still get very chilly. If you have radiation burn take your cream and sun block to keep skin burnt by radiation out of the sun.

> ### REMEMBER
>
> *Skin that has been damaged by radiation from radiotherapy will be extraordinarily sensitive to the sun.*
>
> *Apply sun block and I would also keep that area covered all together. Make sure your swimwear covers the area or you have a kaftan or clothing to keep that area covered and protected.*

Medical Supplies

I always keep medical supplies in my hand luggage because I would never run the risk of my suitcase getting lost and being without vital supplies that may be very hard to get abroad but remember, even with a medical condition the rules for hand luggage contents still apply. No liquids over 100ml, no scissors and so forth.

For me, it is my colostomy bags that are the essential part and would be difficult to get abroad, so I always keep all my colostomy bags in my hand luggage. I pre-cut enough colostomy bags for the flight and then take scissors in my suitcase for when I get there. Scissors I can buy if my case get's lost, medication and colostomy bags will not be so easy. Think about these details.

THE FLIGHT

Although you have access to food and drink on board, I would recommend taking your own. Remember you can't take drinks and certain food through security, but I would buy some once you are through. That way if you need to eat or drink to take medication or ward-off nausea and staff can't get to you at a time you need, it's not a problem.

Think about how long you will be on board for, including possible waiting times either end and work out how many times you will need to take medication, change plasters, whatever it may be and make sure you have enough to see you through the flight. I always take double whatever I think I am going to need, just to be sure.

As I said earlier, if you are on a lot of medication or need constant oxygen, anything like that, check with the airline that there are no restrictions on taking those supplies on board.

ESSENTIAL GUIDE

Before You Book

- ❖ Speak with you oncologist and make sure that they are happy for you to travel and if there is anywhere you should or shouldn't go.
- ❖ Double check that where you want to travel has an equivalent medical system should you need urgent medical attention.
- ❖ Stick to Western European countries that accept the EHIC card.

❖ Avoid anywhere that requires inoculations.
❖ Check travel insurance will cover the destination.
❖ Check your destination can meet any dietary, lifestyle or medical requirements.
❖ Confirm with the airline and destination that you are allowed to take any unusual medication, oxygen tanks, wheelchairs, whatever it is you need, that may not be considered 'standard.'

Before You Go
❖ Get an EHIC card from the NHS.
❖ Check online for local doctors and hospitals in the area.
❖ Relax!

Packing
❖ Take medical notes with you.
❖ Consider highlighting key points in the native language.
❖ Contact details for your UK medical team including your NHS number.
❖ Take at least double the amount of supplies you anticipate needing.
❖ Anything you will need to counteract side effects of treatment.
❖ Sun protection and sun block.

❖ Keep medical supplies in hand luggage but within the legal requirements.

Flight

❖ Take snacks and drinks on board with you.
❖ Ensure you have enough supplies for the flight and possible delays.
❖ Confirm beforehand with the airline you can take any large or unusual medical supplies on-board with you.

USEFUL CONTACTS

www.nhs.uk/NHSEngland?Healthcareabroad/EHIC
www.moneysupermarket.com
www.visitengland.com
www.tripadvisor.com

.

Chapter Eleven

HOW TO SURVIVE AN OCCASION

Time to drink champagne
and dance on the table
- Unknown

A big occasion like Christmas, a wedding, Christening, funeral, or a big birthday party can be difficult enough at the best of times, let alone when you have cancer. Then it can require a lot more planning.

I attended a wedding whilst in the middle of my cancer treatment and I was so stressed by the thought of it, I can't tell you. The wedding venue was two and a half hours away from my house and over three hours away from my hospital. It was going to be the first time that I would be out for the whole day and not within a twenty-minute drive of my house. At least my house was filled with everything I needed. It was also the first occasion I would be attending since having my colostomy bag fitted. It felt like everything was building up for an eventual catastrophe.

I am pleased to report that everything was fine and we had a lovely day but there were some things I found made it easier.

FIRST THINGS FIRST

Don't let the thought of the occasion overwhelm you. Organisation is key when it comes to surviving an occasion with cancer. Obviously I am sure everything will be fine but just like when you are going on holiday - expect the best, prepare for the worst!

Here are a few way's to help you get organised:

Think the day through

In your mind, walk through the day so you can get your head around how the day is expected to play out. For example if you are thinking about Christmas and you are visiting your parents for the day it may be something like:

❖ It's a two-hour drive there and I will need to take painkillers during that time which I need to take with food so I must have some water and fruit with me in the car.

❖ I am going to wear something comfy in the car and change into my outfit when I get there so I will need my outfit packed, including accessories and shoes.

❖ I know we aren't eating until 4pm but I will need a snack to take medication with at lunchtime so I will take some nuts for then.

❖ I need to change plasters at 2pm but we will be having a pre-lunch walk then so I need to make sure I do it before we leave for our walk and take plasters with me.

❖ And so on...

Your Christmas may be completely different to this, but you get the idea. Just run it through you mind or write it down like a schedule so you can get it all straight in your head and you can make sure you have everything you will need.

> ### TOP TIP
> *I find it easy to remember to take medication when I am at home but when I come out of my normal routine I easily forget. Set a reminder on your phone to make sure you don't lose track of what you need to be taking and when.*

If you are attending a wedding or going somewhere where you don't know the schedule, ask the person organising it. Believe me, if it is a wedding, the bride will know exactly when everything is happening and I am sure she will be happy to share details with you so that you can organise your day.

Your Outfit

Think about your outfit and how it is going to work with anything you need to do. If you need to change bandages, make sure they are easily accessible in what you are wearing (or that there will an opportunity to go somewhere to change).

Have your outfit completely ready to go beforehand and that means everything – tights, fascinator, coat, underwear, wig or scarf, literally the whole outfit from top to bottom, including what you need in your handbag. It will save you panicking on the day because you can't find the right denier tights on top of everything else.

Your Handbag

This will be your home away from home, but to save you walking around with a bag that is gong to break your shoulder, I would go for the cute little bag that holds your phone and the bits that you would normally take out with you and then a second bag for medical supplies, change of outfit, whatever it may be.

As a mum I am used to having to pack a changing bag for two children that covers every possible outcome for the day. Now it's about applying those well-honed skills to myself.

TOP TIP

Make sure you have double of the essentials you need. The last thing you want is to be caught short so if you know you will need two painkillers during the time period, take four with you. That way if you get caught in traffic or end up staying later than planned, or any other unexpected circumstance crops up, you know you will be all right.

LOOKING DIFFERENT

It can be difficult attending an occasion when you feel like you don't look like yourself. Whether its weight gain or loss due to medication, you've lost a boob, gained a colostomy or lost your hair, you might feel like it is a huge beacon shouting '*look at me, I have cancer, and it is all we are going to end up talking about, all day!*' I am sure that most of the other guests will be so caught up in whatever the occasion is, they won't even notice but even if they do, I am sure most people are just going to want to make sure you are OK.

That is one of the good things about cancer, most people are very sympathetic, and are just going to want you to have a good time, which was something Alice found when attending a girls weekend away:

I was so excited to be going on a girly weekend for a friend's 40th birthday. It had been planned and booked for months. Then cancer struck __again.__ I was devastated to think I might miss it and so remained determined to go!

It was only a week after my second chemotherapy treatment and I felt awful. I was totally bald and had a PICC line in my arm but there was no stopping me.

I was nervous meeting lots of ladies I'd never met before - what on Earth would they think? But everyone was so lovely. They looked after me and understood when I needed to rest.

That's not to say I didn't get my fair share of looks from other people when we were out at night but I just held my baldhead high and ignored it!

I really enjoyed the weekend and was surprised at how much easier it was than I had anticipated.

*Alice, Hodgkin's Lymphoma, 27
and Ewing's Sarcoma, 37*

KNOW WHEN TO LEAVE

Given the circumstance, I am sure that your friend or loved one will be thrilled that you made the effort and were able to attend their event at all, so don't feel like you have to be the last one on the dance floor. Just do as much as you can and when you start to feel like it is enough, explain to your host that you are starting to feel unwell and have to leave, but you were just so pleased that you could be involved for as long as you were.

I always found when I was getting tired, it would creep up on me and then suddenly I would be beyond exhausted and once I was at that point of exhaustion, I would be knocked out for the next few days and I would then find the pain difficult to stay on top of, so it may be best to leave before that point.

For the wedding I attended, my husband and I went with a clear idea of when we were going to leave. We would stay for the first dance, and then once the festivities got truly underway, we would leave everyone to get on with it and we told the bride and groom before the wedding. Deciding beforehand meant that there were no surprises or awkward conversations. We just had a lovely time and left before it got too much.

LET GO

Having said that, we all need a blow out every now and then. Especially when you are going through something like cancer, so don't feel bad if you do get caught up in the moment and spend the next few days paying for it, just enjoy yourself, you definitely deserve it!

Chapter Twelve

LIFE AFTER CANCER

After a while I looked in the mirror and realised…
Wow. After all those hurts, scars and bruises.
After all of those trials. I did it.
I survived that which was supposed to kill me.
So I straightened my crown.
And walked away. Like a boss.
- Unknown

You've got the all clear. Yay! Congratulations!

So you are skipping through the clouds and singing as you walk down the street and nothing will ever be able to bring you down again, right? The truth is… maybe not.

This is probably a more accurate description of your loved ones reactions when you get the all clear. After however long it has been since your cancer journey

165

began and all your lives have been up in the air, loved ones will be more than ready for life to return to *'normal.'* The only trouble is that this is usually the first opportunity that you will have had to begin processing what has just happened to you.

FINISHING TREATMENT

Finishing treatment is a slightly surreal, strange moment. It is a monumental occasion, but so normal at the same time because it is part of your normal daily routine.

I took my last chemotherapy tablet at home – with champagne (probably not advisable but definitely seemed like a good idea) but two weeks earlier I had my last intravenous chemotherapy session at hospital. I remember thinking I would be so excited when I was finished and leaving the chemotherapy suite. In reality, I felt so ill after four hours of being pumped full of drugs, I was feeling too unwell to be excited about anything.

Emma had her last chemotherapy in hospital and recalls the surreal feeling saying:

I remember at my last chemotherapy appointment expecting some sort of fan-fare, at least an acknowledgement of what I had achieved in finishing treatment, but there was nothing. The nurses just carry on with their jobs. On reflection, of course that's right, other people are still going through their treatment or may not be getting better. I left with such a mix of emotions, it was a very strange feeling and one I hadn't expected.

Emma, Breast Cancer, 27

One my treatment was finished, in a very strange way, I sort of missed hospital. Obviously not the treatment or having cancer but you can go from feeling very protected and insulated by a large team of highly skilled doctors and nurses and then suddenly they all vanish. After so long, it is a very strange sensation and you can feel quite vulnerable, like you are on your own and having to fend for yourself.

THE FIRST YEAR AFTER GETTING THE 'ALL CLEAR'

You may find that the first year after cancer treatment is not quite as easy as you anticipated. I remember being in complete shock, totally unable to process getting the all clear. After years of trying to get a diagnosis and then a year of results turning out to be significantly worse than initially anticipated, I was convinced for months after the 'all clear' that they were going to call me in and say *'sorry, we missed something, it's not over, in fact, it's even worse.'* It's not like breaking an arm and once it's fixed, it's fixed. You keep returning for check-ups and there is the looming possibility of it returning. So don't be surprised if you aren't able to forget about it in the same way that you might with other health conditions, or as quickly as friends and loved ones do.

The result of all this initial uncertainty was that I didn't bounce back from cancer in the way I thought I would. I gave myself a month after my last bout of chemotherapy to feel 'normal' and go back to being a full-time mum but the reality was quite different. I was still feeling the effects of all the medication. I was ill a number of times because of my immune system being so low and I was tired *all the time*.

I really threw myself back into my life straight away. I was keen to feel back in control of my life after feeling that I had missed so much but after a few months I was burnt out. It was one thing feeling better when I had plenty of time to rest, but quite another going back to being a full-time mummy of two toddlers. In the end, I had to take a step back, to evaluate and make some changes, like arranging for my children to go to a childminder for a couple of hours, twice a week so that I could get a little time to rest.

The whole cancer experience left me feeling raw and emotionally drained and the emotional side of my healing did take some time and it took a little while to get used to the changes in my body, being left with a colostomy bag and early menopause.

Please don't think I am sharing this with you to

denigrate the positive news that my cancer has gone. Equally I am not telling you all of this to panic you, but rather let you know that if you are not feeling the elation you were expecting, you are not alone.

Remember, *this too shall pass*. You just need to give yourself a little time.

REMEMBER

Take it one day at a time. This is not an overnight process, it will take time.

Don't rush into anything, listen you your body.

Start to increase what you are doing slowly, allowing for the bad days that inevitably crop up.

MOVING ON

It can be strange after cancer when the biggest emotional breakthroughs (good and bad) come out when you least expect them.

After my mum died, I didn't really cry at any of the big things I was 'meant to' cry at, such as her funeral, but when someone would make it through to live rounds on X-Factor, the first thing they do (after hugging everyone) is call their mum and that would just set something off in me. The fact that they could ring their mum and tell her that something amazing had happened to them and I couldn't would have me in tears every time. Bizarre, but true!

During my last three-month cycle of chemotherapy a friend came to visit me I asked how she was and she said *we are all fine, just plodding along, nothing to report really.* I remember being flabbergasted. I couldn't even think of the last time I had given an answer like that. I remember crying to my husband that I wanted to tell someone that I was just plodding along. After agreeing he would like that too and a few reassurances from that our time would come I left it, still feeling unconvinced.

One day, a while after getting the all clear, a friend text me asking how I was and this is exactly what I wrote back: *'We are okay thanks, just ticking along.'* It probably sounds ridiculous, but for me, it was my post-cancer, breakthrough moment. Finally, things were (relatively) normal.

Don't get me wrong, life is still life, with all its crazy ups and downs, but normal, in a non-cancer kind of way. To be honest, it had probably been like that for a while but finally realising it in my own head felt amazing! And this will happen to you. You will suddenly reach a point where life has become what you want it to be again.

CANCER'S LEGACY

Even though the cancer is gone, certain things remained, like the colostomy, early menopause and HRT, joy! But it's not all bad news.

Most women I have spoken to go through big changes after getting the all clear. I call it a 'shedding of the skin.' It is like drawing a metaphorical line in the sand and creating a 'this is my life *after* cancer' point of distinction.

For me, I wanted to do something new, something that was mine and something that I could be proud of. I wanted to help others who are affected by cancer, which led me to start my blog and fulfil an ambition of writing this book. I wanted to go to university to read Literature and Creative Writing and follow my lifelong dream to be a writer. All of which I am doing and if I am brutally honest, I am not sure I would have made these things happen for myself had I not had a full on face off with my own mortality. I often joke that most people realise they want to spend more time with their family, where as I decided I wanted to spend less time at home, but you know, whatever works!

You will never have your life put so acutely into perspective, than when you think you may lose it, so I actually try and remember that feeling and use it to push myself to do things that I may have flaked out of doing before.

THE ONLY THING HOLDING YOU BACK IS YOU!

When my surgeon discharged me she said, *"We did this so that you could live, so don't live like a patient, make sure you really go out and live."* My initial reaction was that clearly she had no idea just how awful I was feeling, but now I truly understand what she meant. It takes a little time to get out of 'patient' mode and decide how you want your life to be now.

You may feel you have developed as a person and want your future to reflect these changes but straight after cancer you may feel like you don't know how to move forward.

It can be useful to ask yourself a number of questions such as:

❖ What have you always wanted to do, but have always been too afraid to try?
❖ What prevented you from trying?
❖ Often it is our fear of failure that puts us off trying something. What would you do if you couldn't fail?
❖ What would you do if money wasn't a consideration?
❖ Write down a list of things that make you happy. This can include spending time with family, friends, going on holidays, going to the beach, having a meal out, anything.
❖ Write down five things you are passionate about.

This may not give you all the answers to your life, but it may be a good starting point to thinking, what next?

REMEMBER

This is not an overnight process. It may take time. Accept the following year as part of the cancer process.

Just like everything else you have had to endure, you will get through it.

And be even more fabulous at the end!

ABOUT THE AUTHOR

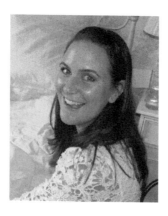

Nicola was diagnosed with an advanced colorectal cancer in 2012, after being told she may not survive, Nicola has been 'all clear' since 2014.

Nicola writes for many health publications on the topics of women's health, cancer and living with an ostomy.

Nicola lives in Hertfordshire with her husband and two children.

www.nicolabourne.wordpress.com
Twitter @njbrn
Facebook @nicolabournewrites

INDEX

177

From my heart to yours,
whoever you are and whatever your story,
I wish you all these best through this time.
With love
Nicola